Transforming Medical
Education for the 21st Century
megatrends, priorities and change

GEORGE R LUEDDEKE
BA OCT MEd PhD
Consultant in Higher and Medical Education Development

Foreword by
MANUEL M DAYRIT
MD MSc
Director, Department of Human Resources for Health
World Health Organization

Commentaries by experts who participated as members of
The Lancet Commission on Education's *Health Professionals for a New Century*

Lord Nigel Crisp
House of Lords, London, UK

Professor Patricia J Garcia MD MPH PhD
Dean, School of Public Health and Administration (FASPA)
Universidad Peruana Cayetano Heredia (UPCH), Lima, Peru

Professor Afaf I Meleis PhD DrPS (Hon) FAAN
Margaret Bond Simon Dean of Nursing
Professor of Nursing and Sociology
University of Pennsylvania School of Nursing
United States

Epilogue by

Ruth Collins-Nakai MD MBA FRCPC MACC
Chair, Canadian Medical Foundation
Ottawa, ON, Canada

Radcliffe Publishing
London • New York

Radcliffe Publishing Ltd
33–41 Dallington Street
London
EC1V 0BB
United Kingdom

www.radcliffepublishing.com

British Library Cataloguing in Publication Data

A catalogue record for this book is available from the British Library.

ISBN-13: 978 184619 969 1

The paper used for the text pages of this book is FSC® certified. FSC (The Forest Stewardship Council®) is an international network to promote responsible management of the world's forests.

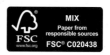

Typeset by Darkriver Design, Auckland, New Zealand
Printed and bound by Hobbs the Printers, Totton, Hants, UK

Contents

Contents

Foreword

In this book, *Transforming Medical Education for the 21st Century: megatrends, priorities and change*, George R Lueddeke looks at two complex issues: the emerging patterns of population health and the challenges to healthcare and the education of the physician of the 21st century.

The author examines present and future issues not only from historical and medical education perspectives but also as an advocate who has a cause to promote and a case to argue. The cause and case are: better healthcare and better education of physicians for the 21st century.

Drawing on national and international reports, the writings of many thinkers and leaders in the field of healthcare, as well as consultations with global experts, the author weaves an extremely informative and thought-provoking discourse about key complex health and social issues we are facing around the globe. Among the many topics in the text, he touches on the changing demographics and inequities in healthcare; medical education priorities, in particular the need for greater integration of inter/trans-professional health education; political and financial concerns; the management of change; the medical profession within the healthcare community. Reflecting directions pursued in numerous reports, he calls for the urgent development of new curriculum frameworks or models for educating future generations of healthcare professionals.

The book comes at a good time for all those concerned with these issues. Just over a year ago, in December 2010, *The Lancet* Commission on education of health professionals for the 21st century launched its groundbreaking report, *Health Professionals for a New Century: transforming education to strengthen health systems in an interdependent world*.[a] This independent initiative, led by a diverse group of 20 commissioners from around the world, adopted a global perspective seeking to advance healthcare by recommending instructional and institutional innovations to nurture a new generation of health professionals who would be better equipped to address present and future health challenges.

Furthermore, in May 2011, Ministers of Health from 193 countries met during the World Health Assembly, and adopted resolution WHA64.6[b] which encouraged all countries to address the pressing issues of health professional education to ensure that the coming generations of health workers were competent to address the challenges of the 21st century within the context of their country's actual needs and aspirations.

Dr Lueddeke is very well placed to write this book as he has worked in both secondary and higher education, including undergraduate and postgraduate medical education, in remote and large urban communities, in both Canada and the United Kingdom. His expertise in educational development has also brought him to different corners of the world.

As both student and expert in education development, the author admits an affinity to 'constructivism'.[c] This is a theory or paradigm which asserts that people construct or create their own knowledge based on personal experiences and hypotheses of the environment. In a very complex world where many health professionals are called to contribute interdependently and in teams to the care of patients and populations, constructivism underpins 'problem-based learning' and 'inter/trans-professional education'.

In Chapter 5, he references the encounter between Alice and the Cheshire cat in *Alice in Wonderland*: 'Which road do I take?', asks Alice. To which the cat replies, 'Where do you want to go?' 'I don't know,' Alice answered. 'Then', said the cat, 'it doesn't matter. If you don't know where you are going, any road will get you there.'

Twenty-first century Alice has a more complex choice before her. Facing her are many roads – radiating, intersecting, winding and passing through unknown territory. Which road to choose?

Paralleling *The Lancet* Commission report, the author argues for fundamental medical/healthcare curriculum changes and opens the door so that readers can consider these within the particular situations they are in. Thus, readers are encouraged to free their imaginations and creative energies towards transforming their own realities. Speaking for myself who has worked in various contexts – healthcare institutions, rural villages, government bureaucracies – with the goal of improving the health of people, this book allows me to look back at my experiences with new eyes and enables me to look at future challenges with imagination and new inspiration.

I am confident that you will find this book an enjoyable, informative and inspiring companion.

Manuel M Dayrit MD MSc
Director, Department of Human Resources for Health
World Health Organization
Geneva, Switzerland
March 2012

References

a Frenk J, Chen L, Bhutta ZA, Cohen J, *et al.* Health professionals for a new century: transforming education to strengthen health systems in an interdependent world. *The Lancet.* 2010; **375**(9721): 1137–8.

b World Health Organization. *Sixty-fourth World Health Assembly closes after passing multiple resolutions* (May 2011). Available at: www.who.int/mediacentre/news/releases/2011/world_health_assembly_20110524/en/index.html (accessed 20 June 2011).

c Learning-Theories.com. *Constructivism.* Available at: www.learning-theories.com/construct ivism.htmlhttp://www.learning-theories.com/ (accessed 15 February 2012).

Commentaries by members of *The Lancet* Commission on Education's *Health Professionals for a New Century*

Global health and professional education

Lord Nigel Crisp, House of Lords, London, United Kingdom

Profound changes in health and healthcare globally over the last 25 years mean that the education of health professionals also needs to change profoundly. There is growing demand for healthcare, and therefore health workers, coming from all round the world. Taken together, this demand far outstrips the current sources of supply. First, the rapidly growing economies, mainly of the East, are facing pressure from their populations to improve public services, particularly healthcare. Second, the ageing and already affluent nations, largely in the West, demand many more health workers to cope with their increasing burden of age-related illnesses and disabilities. Finally, the poorest countries of the world, mostly in sub-Saharan Africa, are struggling to cope with the highest burdens of disease and the lowest numbers of health workers.

Growing demand for health workers, shortages and mal-distribution make up only part of the changes in health underway globally. The world is also experiencing a deep-seated and long-term shift from communicable to non-communicable diseases – with growth in cardiac and vascular diseases, cancer, diabetes and other conditions meaning that throughout the world there are increasing numbers of people living with long-term conditions that grow more debilitating as they age. This change is putting new pressure on older health systems which were designed for a different age when many health problems were acute and short term. The old need for a health system based largely on receiving care from hospitals and health professionals is being replaced by a requirement for a far more diverse and community-based system involving many different people from family to physician and volunteer to trained carer.

These changes in demand and in the nature of that demand are matched by equally marked changes in the way that health workers are now able to be trained, deployed and supported. There is now growing evidence from around the world that new groups of health workers can now safely and effectively do tasks once reserved for more highly trained groups. Moreover, in addition to this 'task shifting' or 'task sharing' new groups such as counsellors, 'peer supporters' and health trainers, for example, are starting to take on roles that were not previously done by anyone at all. There are now many new technologies in the forms of new therapies, new ways of delivering them including the information and communications technologies (ICT) that can support these shifts in how treatment and care are delivered and in how health worker education and training is undertaken.

These global developments set the scene for the radical changes in the education and training of health professionals which are required. Ultimately, it is transformation in how health professionals work and, most fundamental of all, in how they think and how they understand the world that will lead to improvements in health and healthcare.

Other *Lancet* commissioner commentaries

Professor Patricia J Garcia MD MPH PhD, Dean, School of Public Health and Administration (FASPA), Universidad Peruana Cayetano Heredia (UPCH), Lima, Peru

The twenty-first century confronts us with multiple challenges in an interdependent and interconnected world. One of those challenges is the pressing need of transforming the education of health professionals to address global health, and such a task is complex for both developing and developed countries.

Transforming Medical Education for the 21st Century: megatrends, priorities and change is a book that presents a detailed analysis from the author's own extensive experience in medical education and from multiple international reports and documents from experts in health education and healthcare. It relates very much to the work of *The Lancet* Commission on Education's *Health Professionals for a New Century* in which I had the opportunity to participate as a commissioner.

Dr Lueddeke explores in his book a particularly interesting view of the drivers of change in medical education and how the lessons learned in the past could guide the future approaches to education and includes a systemic view in which the interactions between physicians and patients have to be considered in the conceptualisation of medical education.

What I really like about Dr Lueddeke's book is that he presents not only new concepts or ideas but also diverse examples of ways to start this 'transformation' in countries, irrespective of their location in the North or in the South. This book will be of interest to all, because it offers more than just a discussion of changes in the education of health professionals; it offers suggestions to real enabling actions.

Professor Afaf I Meleis PhD DrPS (Hon) FAAN, Margaret Bond Simon Dean of Nursing, University of Pennsylvania School of Nursing, Philadelphia, PA, USA

Fortified by scientific revolutions, the increasing engagement of healthcare consumers in their own care, technological innovations, ease in communication through social media, vast movements of populations from rural to urban settings and from country to country, increasing expectations for integration of knowledge and mounting evidence that teamwork in healthcare produces safe and quality care, educators will increasingly find it imperative to cross disciplines and transcend countries.

Interdisciplinarity and interprofessionalism are the present and the future in educating healthcare professionals and in liberating healthcare teams from adhering to archaic structures that prepared physicians more for leadership and less for team membership, more for cure than prevention and more for individual care than community care. In this well-constructed volume on medical education, Dr Lueddeke begins with the explicit recommendations of the spirit of *The Lancet* report and honours the implicit values of 'teamwork', global reciprocity and quality care that goes beyond cure and active lifestyle needs, putting families and communities at the core of care and breaking interprofessional barriers. This book is another milestone in progress towards transforming medical education from the tenets that dominated it in the 20th century to those that reflect the proposed global healthcare reforms for the 21st century.

Rightly or wrongly, medicine has been conceived as the leader in healthcare. Therefore, devoting a volume for how to transform the education of physicians to become more collaborative, holistic, integrative, family and community-based and more inclusive of lifestyle continuum, is essential. While some may argue that the transformation of education requires a volume that encompasses the education of other essential members in the healthcare team, such as professionally-educated nurses, devoting a volume to medical education is a giant step forward that could inspire others to devote similar writings to other professions.

Interprofessional education needs to benefit from the wisdom of the different professions. As one example, nurses, the largest healthcare workforce in the world, and front-line healthcare providers, are integral partners for creating and translating best practices for quality care and for shaping the future of interprofessional healthcare education. The nursing discipline has a unique, patient-centred, holistic approach in looking at global healthcare challenges. Nursing's mission is focused on providing the evidence for preventing illness, promoting health, enhancing quality of life and supporting self-care of populations, as well as using a human justice and equity framework in providing access to healthcare and to better quality of life. Therefore, nurses are vital in promoting teamwork and collaboration to ensure the implementation of *The Lancet* Commission recommendations and make a positive impact in the health and well-being of the world.

Integrating transformative curricula is a next step in progress towards achieving *The Lancet* report recommendations. A new era in interdependent and global professional education requires reforms in admission, accreditation, exploitation of the powers of IT learning, breaking the silos between professions, adoption of competency-based curriculum, expansion to academic systems, forming of global health profession networks and nurturing a culture of critical inquiry, in addition to the integration of knowledge generated by the different professions.

Implementation of *The Lancet* report recommendations, and the exquisite, thoughtful, team-based, population-focused and globally-driven chapters in this volume, requires flexibility in curriculum design by medical educators – along with all other health/social care professions – and an embodied understanding of the tremendous changes in the health and social care needs of populations.

It will require transformation in a paradigm that focused on illness and cure to one that puts the healthcare utiliser's needs within the context of their socio-cultural and community contexts. It will require a total reconceptualisation of individualised, medically-based care to a personalised collaborative learner and community-based care. It will also be necessary to pay particular attention to the interconnection between the educational and health systems and to population and labour markets to accurately assess health professionals' needs and supply and demand needs. In this seminal and ground-breaking volume written by this forward looking and future making author, the reader will find a framework for the aims of revitalising medical education as well as guidelines that operationalise these aims into specific curricular models, making it feasible for faculty to use in transforming didactic, clinical training and the pedagogies used in teaching.

This book could be transformative and a turning point in medical education specifically and healthcare education generally. It is a step in the right direction and should be required reading for educators, students/trainees and managers in medicine, nursing, public health and other health/social care professions. It is a driver and facilitator in advancing progress in interprofessional education.

We are at the dawn of a new era in the education of health professionals, prompted by the landmark report on *Health Professionals for a New Century: transforming education to strengthen health systems in an interdependent world.* This volume is a vital catalyst and facilitator to enhance progress in this new era.

Preface

This book originated from lectures, seminars and conference presentations given over several years to incoming medical students, postgraduate trainees and medical educators in Canada, the United Kingdom, the United States and Sri Lanka. I was motivated to write about the need to reconceptualise and transform medical education while preparing a manuscript on the history of medical education and the rise of the specialties in Britain, written primarily for busy medical students, including prospective ones, parents or guardians, postgraduate trainees, healthcare educators or anyone else who may be interested in seeing the 'bigger picture'.

In essence, the book builds on and complements the latter text and explores how medicine and medical education may evolve in the coming decades. Written for medical educators, practitioners, policymakers and healthcare professionals generally, this book seeks to understand why many national and international bodies or committees are calling for major improvements in both undergraduate and postgraduate medical education. In addition, from an educational developer perspective, the text aims to share approaches for conceptualising and designing future medical curricula and managing change, while recognising current constraints and uncertainties.

More specifically, discussions focus on attempting to answer the following questions:

- What are the key drivers of change and what impact are they having (or will they have) on patient care?
- What are national and international reviews telling us about their medical education priorities?
- What common themes are emerging from national and international studies?
- What emerging principles may underpin medical education curricula in the future?
- What have we learned about enacting change in medical education in the past and what approaches to change management may be useful to consider in future?

- How is the 'physician–patient' contract changing and what impact could this have on conceptualising and managing medical education?
- How can we translate future visions and recommended reforms into reality on the ground?
- What educational models are emerging that encourage interprofessional and transprofessional learning in medical education?
- How can population growth, consumption and interdependency be harmonised in the twenty-first century?
- Finally, what sense of purpose or common aspirations may cohere students, trainees, healthcare professionals and policymakers generally in order to optimise patient safety and quality of care?

George R Lueddeke
March 2012

About the author

George Lueddeke BA OCT MEd PhD is an educational consultant in higher and medical education. In his early career he was a secondary school teacher and later worked in post-secondary education establishing programmes for English-speaking, francophone and Native Cree communities in Ontario and northern Canada communities. He has held posts in educational and organisational development, management, research and teaching in both Canada and the United Kingdom and has led a number of national and provincial projects.

Specialising in higher and medical education, educational development and change management, he has also conducted workshops and seminars in Canada, the United States, the United Kingdom and Sri Lanka as well as for visiting groups (e.g. from China, Mexico, Malaysia, Japan). Also over the years a consultant education adviser with the Kent, Surrey & Sussex Postgraduate Deanery in London, he was previously senior lecturer in medical education at Southampton's School of Medicine and received a Vice Chancellor's Teaching Excellence Award in 2006.

His main research interests are focused on the nature and philosophy of curriculum, culturally diverse and inter/trans-professional educational practices, the professionalisation of teaching, the management of change and innovation in higher education generally and socio-historical perspectives on medicine and healthcare in particular in developed and developing countries. He is the author of a number of Canadian provincial studies, occupational analyses and institutional texts on teaching and has written numerous articles on these themes for international journals.

He has been a keynote speaker and presented at international conferences and seminars on change management, curriculum planning and historical perspectives on medical education, including, inter alia, by invitation, sessions for the Wessex Postgraduate Deanery and the Education Directorate of the General Medical Council in the United Kingdom.

He lives in the New Forest, Hampshire, in the United Kingdom, with his wife, Jill and family members.

Acknowledgements

First, I wish to express my sincere gratitude and appreciation to my colleagues in the Faculty of Medicine and the Faculty of Health Sciences at the University of Southampton and fellow professionals at the Kent, Surrey & Sussex Postgraduate Deanery in London. Colleagues in these committed and excellent organisations allowed me to experience 'medical' education and to contribute to initiatives that always have as their main goal the enhancement of the student or trainee learning experience. Without their ongoing support and opportunities for engagement in many innovative and exciting professional and educational developments, this book would not have been possible.

For giving constructive and encouraging feedback on the manuscript, I am indebted to Dr Lincoln Chen, president of the China Medical Board, Professor Julio Frenk, dean of Harvard's School of Public Health, and Dr Catherine Michaud, consultant with the China Medical Board.

I would also like to sincerely express my appreciation to Dr Manuel M Dayrit, director of the Department of Human Resources for Health at the World Health Organization, for raising my awareness of the critical issues facing developing countries and for contributing the Foreword to this book. For writing book commentaries I wish to thank the distinguished *Lancet* commissioners Lord Nigel Crisp, UK House of Lords and former chief executive of the NHS and permanent secretary at the Department of Health (2000–06); Professor Patricia J Garcia, professor of the School of Public Health at Cayetano Heredia University, Peru, and former chief of the Peruvian National Institute of Health (2006–08); and Professor Afaf I Meleis, Margaret Bond Simon Dean of Nursing at the University of Pennsylvania and director of the School's WHO Collaborating Centre for Nursing and Midwifery Leadership. In addition, gratitude is extended to Dr Ruth Collins-Nakai, former president of the Canadian Medical Association and chair of the Canadian Medical Foundation, for writing an epilogue.

Many people contributed to this book by reading chapters and sections, answering questions, raising issues and offering creative suggestions. For providing detailed and exceptionally helpful feedback, I would especially like to express my gratitude to Dr Jacalyn Duffin, physician and medical historian at Queen's University, Canada; Dr Brenda Zierler, professor of the Department of Biobehavioral Nursing and Health Systems at the University of Washington, United States; Dr Shafik Dharamsi, assistant professor in medicine and associate in residence, Liu Institute for Global Issues, University of British Columbia, Canada; and Dr Andrew Perry, advanced trainee, emergency medicine and clinical associate lecturer, University of Adelaide, Australia.

My personal thanks also go to Paul Buckley, director of education at the General Medical Council, UK; Dr Andrew Pesce, former president of the Australian Medical Association; Dr Norman Carr, principal clinical teaching fellow and honorary consultant pathologist, University of Southampton; Professor Loren Cordain, Department of Health and Exercise Science, Colorado State University, United States; Professor Brian Hodges, vice-president Education, University Health Network and professor, Department of Psychiatry, University of Toronto, Canada; Dr Ed Miller, dean of the US Johns Hopkins Medical School, United States; Professor Roger Bootle, managing director of Capital Economics; Pam Jackson, curriculum coordinator for Interprofessional Learning for the University of Southampton and Portsmouth University, UK; Professor Russell Mannion, professor of health systems at the Health Services Management Centre, University of Birmingham, UK; and Dr Rob Marchbanks, Neurological Physics Group, Department of Medical Physics, University Hospital Southampton NHS Foundation Trust, UK.

For acknowledging the potential contribution of this work to medicine and medical education, I thank Dr George Thibault, president of the US Macy Foundation; Dr Sarkis Meterissian, associate dean of postgraduate medical education and professional affairs at McGill University, Canada; Mrs Linda de Cossart CBE, director of medical education at Chester NHS Foundation Trust, UK; Dr Della Fish, professor of education at the University of Wales, UK; Professor Debra Humphris, pro-vice chancellor, education, and Dr Chris Stephens, university director and associate dean, Faculty of Medicine, University of Southampton, UK; Dean Director Dr David Black, professor Zoë Playdon, head of education and Dr Pam Shaw, former deputy head of education, Kent, Surrey & Sussex Postgraduate Deanery, UK; Professor Sir Richard Thompson, president and Winnie Wade, director of education at the Royal College of Physicians, London, UK; Dr David Blumenthal, director, US Institute for Health Policy; David Naylor, president of the University of Toronto, Ontario, Canada; Professor Geoff McColl, director of the Medical Education Unit at the Melbourne Medical School, Australia; Professor John Bligh, dean of medical education, Dr Lynn Morouxe, director of education, School of Medicine, Cardiff University; Dr James Le Fanu, columnist for *The Daily* and *Sunday Telegraph*; Peter Sharp, chief executive, Dr Graham Willis, head of Analytics, Meena Mahil, and Hannah Darvill at the UK Centre for Workforce Intelligence (CfWI); Robbert Duvivier, medical educationalist and member of the Faculty Council at Maastricht University, Netherlands; Dr Richard Horton, editor-in chief of *The Lancet*; Professor George Lewith, UK College of Medicine; Dr Patrick Kelley, director, Boards on Global Health and African Science Academy Development, Institute of Medicine, US.

I owe a special note of appreciation to Dr Kevin Eva, a fellow Canadian and editor of the highly regarded journal *Medical Education*, who suggested that I turn a rather lengthy journal article into a book. I also wish to express my personal thanks to Gillian Nineham, director of publishing at Radcliffe Publishing along with her highly professional and supportive team, including Tanya Dean, Jamie Etherington, Ushma Mistry, Alice French, Rachel Inger, Martin Hill, and Camille Lowe at Undercover project management. I also extend my appreciation to my wife, Jill, for her constructive suggestions and allowing me the 'space' (sometimes reluctantly!) to write this book and to Daniel Crouchman and Alexander Carr for their technical and personal support ('sounding boards') while writing the manuscript.

I am also grateful for permission to reproduce original images or artwork from *The Lancet* Commission report *Health Professionals for a New Century: transforming education to strengthen health systems in an interdependent world*, courtesy of Professor Julio Frenk, dean of the Harvard School of Public Health, and Dr Lincoln Chen, president of the China Medical Board; an exhibit and graphs from the report *Mirror, Mirror On The Wall: how the performance of the U.S. healthcare system compares internationally: 2010 Update*, courtesy of Dr Karen Davis, president of the Commonwealth Fund; use of an infographic showing 2009 comparative country health data, courtesy of *National Geographic*; world overweight and obesity graphs, courtesy of the National Obesity Observatory; interprofessional learning unit schedule (11 healthcare programmes), courtesy of Pam Jackson, interprofessional earning coordinator, University of Southampton and Portsmouth University; and the figure showing industrial versus information age medicine, courtesy of Professor Tricia Greenhalgh, joint lead Global Health, Policy and Innovation Unit, Centre for Primary Care and Public Health, Barts and The London School of Medicine and Dentistry (adapted from T Ferguson. Consumer health informatics. *Healthcare Forum J* 1995: Jan–Feb.: 28–33); synoptical reference to William Bridge's *Managing Transitions*, courtesy of Susan Bridges, president of William Bridges and Associates, Larkspur, California; image of earth from the outer edge of the solar system, courtesy of Jody Russell, Media Resource Centre, Nasa Johnson Space Centre, Houston, Texas, US.

Readers are asked to note that the ideas contained in this publication are my own and are by no means shared by all chapter reviewers or contributors or by any of the institutions for which I have worked.

Figures and tables

Figures

Tables

For Jill, my wife and soul mate
David, Jennifer, Sara, Christina, Katrina, Lisa and John,
their partners and families –
with love and thanks.

The best way to predict the future is to create it.
—Professor Peter Drucker (1909–2005)

Introduction

Although Charles Dickens's *A Tale of Two Cities*[1] was published in 1859 and is set during the French Revolution in the late eighteenth century, the paradoxical and eloquent opening paragraph could easily apply to the beginning years of the twenty-first century:

> It was the best of times, it was the worst of times, it was the age of wisdom, it was the age of foolishness, it was the epoch of belief, it was the epoch of incredulity, it was the season of Light, it was the season of Darkness, it was the spring of hope, it was the winter of despair, we had everything before us, we had nothing before us, we were all going direct to Heaven, we were all going direct the other way – in short, the period was so far like the present period, that some of its noisiest authorities insisted on its being received, for good or for evil, in the superlative degree of comparison only.

With two world wars, countless conflicts, terrorism, pandemics, severe recessions, poverty and socio-economic disparities, throughout the twentieth century people certainly experienced 'the worst of times'. But, unlike in Dickens's era, the twentieth century also witnessed major improvements in the standard of living, life expectancy, transport and communication, science, nutrition, education and, of course, medicine generally. Regrettably, however, the majority of people worldwide (well over 5 billion of an estimated world population of 7 billion) have not yet had the opportunity to benefit from many of these achievements, and they continue to face many hard 'winters of despair'.

In a cautiously optimistic article, 'Why most things keep getting better – and a few get worse',[2] economist Roger Bootle reminds us that, because of gradual accumulation of capital and technology, living standards have improved continually since the Industrial Revolution. Although there are many threats to our way of life, he suggests there are two factors that 'give hope to the future': the first is that countries such as China and India that have for the past 200 years relied extensively, for economic reasons, on Europe – and, more recently, the United States and Japan – will increasingly contribute to human knowledge and from these countries the West can learn, for example, how 'to economise the use of scarce resources'. The second factor is the potential of technology – in particular, the importance of the internet and its capacity to 'speed up technological progress'. However, as with most new ways of doing things, Bootle observes there are also many downsides to these 'high tech' developments, at least until consumers demand 'a better-quality version', a scenario that may resonate today with respect to patient care.

Ian Morris, archaeologist and professor of classics and history at Stanford University in the United States, in *Why the West Rules – For Now: the patterns of history, and what they reveal about the future*,[3] tells us that 'on average, all over the world, people are 50% bigger than in 1900' and that the human body has changed more in the past 100 years than it did in the previous 100 000 years. While this evolution will likely continue, some changes may not be for the better. Arguing convincingly in *Tomorrow's People: how 21st century technology is changing the way we think and feel*,[4] and in subsequent articles, well-known neuropharmacologist Baroness Susan Greenfield cautions that the 'rewiring' of the human brain ('mind change'), with technology becoming 'increasingly bio-dominated', could have a major impact on the human condition – possibly 'shortening attention spans, encouraging instant gratification and causing a loss of empathy', the latter possible outcome being particularly worrisome in health and social care. Considered collectively, Professor Morris predicts we can expect 'new ways of living, fighting, working, thinking and loving, new ways of being born, growing old, and dying'.[3]

Medical advances will hopefully continue to have mostly positive impacts on our lives. William Haseltine, chairman and chief executive officer of US company Human Genome Sciences, claims that both regenerative and rejuvenative medicine will be important in the twenty-first century. He suggests the first half will be 'dominated by the use of human genes, proteins, antibodies and cells to replace, repair and restore what has been damaged by disease, injured by trauma or worn by time', while the second 'will be even better', with the 'introduction of atomic scale protheses to repair and restore human body function'. If these developments materialise, human lives and lifestyle generally will be fundamentally transformed during this century.[5]

These and other directions in society generally, and healthcare specifically, will greatly influence the education and training of health and social care workers across the globe. Ensuring that this training is of the highest standard – including the most recent medical advancements and research findings – and that it matches population needs is fundamentally crucial to the welfare and well-being of patient care and the global society as a whole. Moreover, as discussed in this book, the importance of strengthening inter/trans-professional learning and working has been highlighted in recent national and international reports investigating medical education. With a more demanding public – calling for more choice, access, convenience and quality care – the pressure on governments for greater accountability, competition and control of professionals will likely grow.

In the more immediate term, reconceptualising of healthcare syllabi may also be necessary as changing expectations and relationships, including the shift from hospital to community care with heightened attention on the elderly and primary care, take hold. Given emerging practice, curricula may need to become more role explicit, paying particular attention to changing patient demographics and requirements, curriculum structures and affordability of training. Moreover, to optimise learner and supervisor support, medical educators may be tasked with improving curricula documentation by enhancing accessibility and curriculum integration (e.g. curative and preventive medicine) as well as supporting individual learner needs through more flexible delivery and mobility.

Referring to the UN Millennium Declaration,[6] signed on 8 September 2000, the lead authors of *Who's Got the Power? Transforming health systems for women and children*[7] pose the fundamental question 'What kind of world do we want to live in?' While the declaration's 'goals are lofty' and '[i]ts hopes are high', the authors express apprehension about whether countries will take the goals set out seriously.

> The global community, particularly those who hold power in countries both rich and poor, have the courage to make the decisions, to challenge the status quo, to guide the transformative change necessary to advance this vision. Will those whose lives and health depend on these actions have the space, the leverage, and the will to demand and ensure that they do?[7]

Echoing the authors of the report, perhaps our most difficult or problematic question this century is finding consensus on where society wants or needs to go. William (Bill) Joy, American computer scientist and co-founder of Sun Microsystems, sharpens the urgency of the query by asking: 'If we could agree, as a species, what we wanted, where we are headed, and why, then we would make our future much less dangerous – then we might understand what we can and should relinquish.'[8] Surely, self-preservation is not one of these.

Key drivers of change

THE BEGINNING DECADES OF THE TWENTY-FIRST CENTURY HAVE BEEN unsettling. Worldwide, many have been affected by natural disasters, terrorism, wars, the Arab Spring, drought and famine, pandemics and financial turbulence. Faced with unprecedented demographic changes and corresponding health and social care needs, coupled with the incapacity to sustain these financially, governments are having to make tough decisions that may have adverse effects on the quality of life not only of today's generation but also of the next. Along with services such as education, social care, the police and the military, healthcare has become a major area for scrutiny, as both societal expectations and costs to meet them have risen sharply over the past few decades. Addressing these urgent issues – key drivers of change – may no longer simply be a matter of 'doing things better' (evolutionary change) or more efficiently but, rather, learning how to 'do better things' (innovation).

Changing demographics and redefining health priorities

A significant contributing factor to the present unease over healthcare in the Western world is the ageing population. For example, it is estimated that in the European Union '[the] number of people aged 65 or over in the total population will increase from 84.6 million in 2008 to 151.5 million in 2060, and those 'aged 80 or over will almost triple from 21.8 million in 2008 to 56.4 million in 2060'.[9]

Advances in medicine, diet and sanitation in the last 100 years are continuing to make a difference in life expectancy with improved sanitary conditions likely to be one of the leading contributors (*see* Figure 1.1). However, while life expectancy has increased, it is debatable whether or not the quality of life has improved for the majority of populations. Although there have been many achievements, mostly in developed nations, in the light of an ageing population and poor lifestyle

Achievements
- smallpox
- Guinea worm disease
- polio

Greatly reduced (developed countries only)
- diptheria
- typhoid fever
- tuberculosis
- whooping cough
- pneumonia
- influenza
- bronchitis
- scarlet fever
- cholera
- malaria

Major health issues in the twenty-first century[11]
- heart attacks and strokes
- pneumonia
- AIDS (HIV)

- pulmonary diseases
- cancer
- obesity
- diabetes
- malnutrition
- Alzheimer's/Parkinson's
- mental well-being/depression
- substance abuse
- rheumatoid arthritis
- MRSA/*C. difficile*
- pandemics
- antibiotic resistance
- diet and nutrition
- ethnic considerations
- 'medicalisation' of society
- preventable medical errors
- widening social disparities
- matching medical education to population needs
- inter/trans-professional teamworking
- critical shortages of health workers in rural and remote areas

FIGURE 1.1 Patterns of disease (from the nineteenth to the twenty-first century)[10]

choices, we are seeing an increase in treatment of chronic health problems. These problems include senile dementia, obesity, diabetes, cardiovascular conditions, alcoholism, drug abuse and cancers.[10]

In developing countries, the World Health Organization (WHO) predicts that by 2030 AIDS/HIV-related deaths will soar from 2.8 million in 2011 to 6.5 million worldwide, and tobacco-related deaths will increase from over 5 million in 2011 to about 8.3 million by that time … Unchanged in the last few decades, heart attacks, strokes, pneumonia, AIDS (HIV) and pulmonary diseases remain the five top health problems.[11]

And, while there has been progress in some areas toward achieving the Millennium Development Goals,[6] 'it has been uneven'. The number of people who are currently undernourished and living in extreme poverty has risen to over 1.4 billion. Progress in achieving gender equality and the empowerment of women has also been 'sluggish', according to the UN Millennium Development Goals report 2010.[12]

It is unfortunate that the arguments put forth by the lead authors of *Who's Got the Power? Transforming health systems for women and children*,[7] issued in 2005, still seem equally relevant seven years later. The report, focusing on the urgent needs of women and children, prepared by a group of leading experts, sought to address the challenges 'posed by high rates of maternal mortality, continued child deaths due to preventable illness, enormous unmet need for sexual and reproductive health services, and weak and fragmented health systems'. In their deliberations, the authors point out that, while technical interventions 'are generally simple and low-tech, even cost-effective', most of the 'world's population do not benefit from them'. For 'hundreds of millions of people', most of whom live in sub-Saharan Africa and southeast Asia, 'the health systems are in crisis – ranging from serious dysfunction to total collapse'.

Further, the authors conclude that 'behind the failure of health systems lies a deeper, structural crisis symbolised by a development programme that permits its own glowing rhetoric to convert the pressure for real change into a managerial programme of technical adjustments', resulting in 'a terrible disconnect between the dominant development models and prescriptions and the brutal realities that people face in their daily lives'.

The authors of the report place responsibility for this chasm squarely on the disconnect or delinking of 'mainstream development practice … from the broader economic and political forces that have generated a level of inequity, exclusion, divisiveness, and insecurity that will not be bottled or stashed away … [t]oo many bold attempts have been neutralised', and 'the damage now lies exposed'. While the solutions are partly technical, the main response called for by the 189 heads of state and government who signed the Millennium Declaration is 'deeply and fundamentally political'.

> It is about access to and the distribution of power and resources within and between countries; in the structures of global governance; and in the intimate space of families, households and communities.[7]

Social determinants of health

On a global scale, the authors of the WHO-commissioned report *Closing the Gap in a Generation: health equity through action on the social determinants of health*,[13] draw our attention to the fact that life chances of children depend on where they are born. For example, '[i]n Japan or Sweden they can expect to live more than 80 years; in Brazil, 72 years; India, 63 years; and in one of several African countries, fewer than fifty years'. Further, they report '[w]ithin countries, the difference in life chances are dramatic and are seen in all countries – even the richest,' with the poorest, unsurprisingly, evidencing high levels of illness and premature mortality. The main message of the Commission on Social Determinants of Health is that '[i]t does not have to be this way and it is not right that it is'. It also believes that '[t]he global community can put this right but it will take urgent and sustained action, globally, nationally, and locally'. Arguing for a new approach to development, the Commission advises that economic growth 'without appropriate social policies to ensure reasonable fairness in the way its benefits are distributed brings little benefit to health equity'. Further, the Commission observes that the 'high burden of illness' arises 'in large part because of the conditions in which people are born, grow, live, work, and age' – 'the consequences of poor social policy. Its main recommendations for 'closing the gap in a generation' are to 'improve the conditions of daily life; tackle the inequitable distribution of power, money, and resources; and, measure and understand the problem and assess the impact of action'.

The Commission raises a final question: 'Is closing the health gap in a generation feasible?' Its two answers provide a succinct choice for 'the whole of government, civil society and local communities, business, global fora, and international agencies':

> If we continue as we are, there is no chance at all. If there is a genuine desire to change, if there is a vision to create a better and fairer world where people's life chances and their health will no longer be blighted by the accident of where they happen to be born, the colour of their skin, or the lack of opportunities afforded to their parents, then the answer is: we could go a long way towards it.

The report's final word is just as compelling: 'Reducing health inequities is, for the Commission on Social Determinants of Health, an ethical imperative. Social injustice is killing people on a grand scale.'

Obesity: 'a diet to disaster'[14]

Closely linked to the social determinants of health are the growing rates of obesity and malnutrition in developing countries. Obesity, which simply means the accumulation of excess fat, has been defined clinically as individuals who have a body mass index (BMI) of 30 or greater. Current estimates are that if someone's BMI is less than 18.5 he or she is underweight; if it is between 18.5 to 24.9 the person has a healthy weight; if between 25 to 29.9, he or she is overweight, and over 29.9, the individual is considered obese.

To calculate body mass index, we divide an individual's weight by his or her height squared [weight (kg) / (height (m) × height (m)] or (BMI = kg/m^2).[15]

So, someone who is 1.70 m and weighs 60 kg has a BMI of $60/(1.7 \times 1.7) = 20.8$.

This person is in the normal category. On the other hand, using imperial (non-metric) measures, someone who is 5'6" (5'6" = 66") and weighs 160 lb has a BMI of 160 / (66 × 66) × 703 = 25.8, and this person is in the overweight category.

Increasing at 'an alarming rate' since the 1980s, 'across OECD [Organisation for Economic Co-operation and Development] countries, one in two adults is currently overweight [BMI = 25 to 29.9] and 1 in 6 is obese [BMI = over 29.9]'. The rate of overweight people is projected to increase by a further 1% per year for the next 10 years in some countries (*see* Figure 1.2).[16]

A 2010 report entitled *Obesity and the Economics of Prevention: fit not fat*[17] released by the OECD projects that 75% of us will be overweight by 2020.

Figure 1.2 shows 'the current levels of obesity and predicted future figures if we continue at our current pace'.[17]

Obesity rates are highest in the United States,[18] where three out of four people are projected by the OECD to be overweight or obese within 10 years, and Mexico, where 'individual prevention programmes could avoid up to 47 000 deaths from chronic diseases every year'.[17] Obesity rates are lowest in Japan and Korea, 'but have been growing virtually everywhere, and have impacted negatively on the lives of children'. According to WHO data, one in three of the world's kids will become overweight and will thereby also have a shorter lifespan. 'Severely obese people die 8–10 years sooner than those of normal-weight, similar to

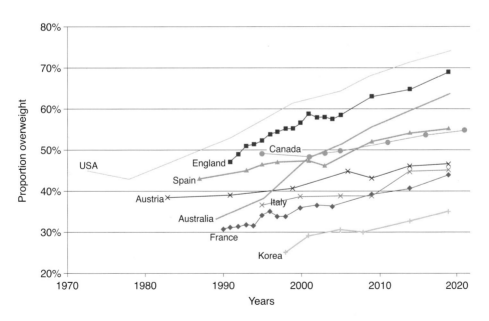

FIGURE 1.2 Past and projected future overweight rates in selected countries of the Organisation for Economic Co-operation and Development

smokers, and they are more likely to develop diseases such as diabetes, cardio-vascular disease and cancer.'[17]

Figure 1.3 lists adult obesity rates across the world. In Canada, about one in four adults is obese, according to 2007–09 data.[19] In Germany, obesity 'has been increasingly cited as a major health issue in recent years'.[20] Britain's adult obesity rate is 23%, twice that of France, and it is the highest in Europe. In England, rates have increased faster than in most countries. Two out of three men are overweight and one in four people are obese in the United Kingdom.[21] Obesity rates in Japan, South Korea and Sweden are low, relative to most other countries. 'One person in 10 is obese in Sweden, but over 1 in 2 men and 1 in 3 women are overweight'.[17]

In Australia, where 'obesity has overtaken smoking as the leading cause of premature death and illness', 'more than 17 million are overweight or obese'. It is predicted that '[i]f weight gain continues at current levels, by 2020, 80% of all Australian adults and a third of all children will be overweight or obese.'[22] A shocking new statistic comes from China where it is estimated that a third of its population, over 429 million, 'are now overweight or obese – a prime candidate for heart disease and diabetes'.[23]

Taken together, the Australian conclusions speak for most nations that '[o]n the basis of present trends we can predict that by the time they reach the age of 20 our kids will have a shorter life expectancy than earlier generations simply because of obesity'.[22]

Figure 1.3 indicates that the countries with the greatest number of obese adults reside in the United States (c. 33.8%) and Mexico (30.0%), followed closely by Scotland, New Zealand, Australia, Canada, Northern Ireland and England. These figures are several years old, and it is probable that they have been rising since.

In a disturbing article on obesity, 'The children eating their way to cancer: expert warns of obesity timebomb', Professor Kathy Pritchard-Jones is quoted say-ing 'thousands will die if parents and ministers do not take the childhood obesity epidemic more seriously' and that '[o]besity is linked to cancers including those of the kidney, breast, colon, liver and prostate. It can also lead to heart disease, stroke and type 2 diabetes, and experts warn the rising tide of these diseases could bankrupt the National Health Service [NHS]'.[14] Further, Figure 1.4, appearing in the same article, expands the types of illnesses that can be triggered by excess fat. Figures 1.5 and 1.6 offer a stark reminder that overweight and obese chil-dren are becoming prime candidates for many of these illnesses or conditions. Unsurprisingly, the countries with the highest number of overweight and obese children in most cases mirror the general adult population with the United States and Mexico leading the way. Poor diet and lack of exercise are the likely causes.

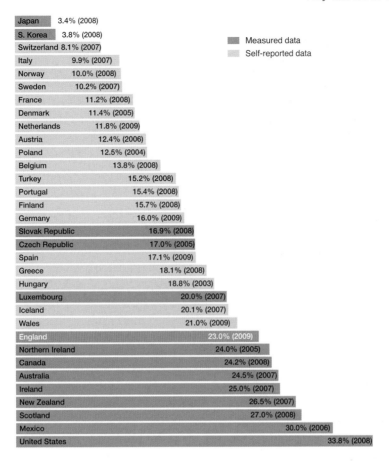

FIGURE 1.3 Adult obesity prevalence: latest available data[24]

A diet to disaster
- Excess fat around the stomach can trigger breast and prostate cancer. This 'adipose tissue', as it is known, causes dangerous changes in the balance of hormones.
- Fat has also been implicated in liver, pancreatic and kidney cancers.
- Obesity reduces the body's level of cytokines, chemicals that can protect against cancer. This is thought to be a factor in colon cancer. A diet low in fresh fruit but high in red meat can also increase the risk of colon cancer.
- Obesity may lead to cancer of the oesophagus (the gullet or food pipe). A larger stomach can exert pressure on the oesophagus. This causes intestinal acid to rise up, which can alter the tissue and make it more likely to develop tumours.

FIGURE 1.4 'A diet to disaster'[14]

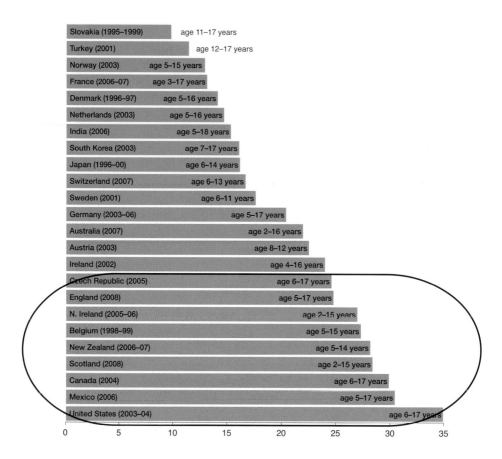

FIGURE 1.5 Prevalence of overweight (including obesity) for boys in selected countries (based on measured height and weight, showing measurement (as a percentage) and age group measured)[24]

According to the OECD, prevention – 'combining health promotion campaigns, government regulation and family doctors counselling'[14] is the key to reducing obesity rates. However, while these strategies are constructive at national levels, including considerably more emphasis in medical education and training, they need to be focused on the community level – a theme that reverberates throughout this book.

Among the strategies that the US Centres for Disease Control and Prevention are 'promoting are making healthy food more available, promoting more choices of healthy foods, promoting breast-feeding, encouraging physical activity and creating sites in communities that support physical activity'.[25] Established in 1986 and with 31 member associations in 33 countries, the European Association for the Study of Obesity aims to 'improve the quality of obesity education in Europe' and 'develop a coherent approach to obesity management throughout Europe'. One

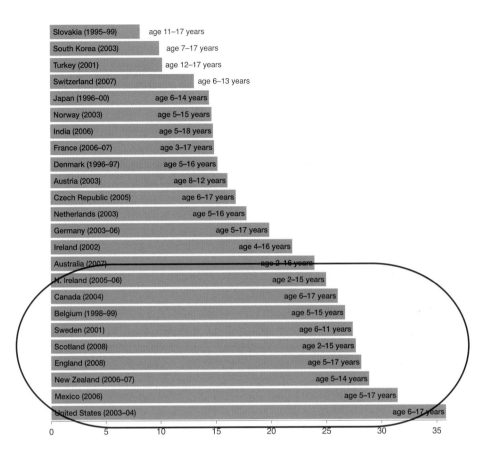

FIGURE 1.6 Prevalence of overweight (including obesity) for girls in selected countries (based on measured height and weight, showing measurement (as a percentage) and age group measured)[14]

of its key strategies is 'to organise educational workshops and sessions around Europe on subjects that are proposed by National Associations'.[26]

Overall, studies[17] have shown that taking 'a multi-stakeholder approach',[27] 'encompassing not just epidemiology and economics but others such as political economy and cognitive science'[28] is the way forward in responding to the obesity crises globally, including:

- physician-dietitian counselling in schools
- fiscal measures ('altering the prices of healthy and unhealthy foods, regulation of food advertising to children and mandatory nutrition labelling'[17])
- worksite intervention
- physician counselling.

Unfortunately, negative measures often driven by profit margins are compromising these positive measures. For example, society seems to be caving in to 'bulging bodywork', as 'car makers are gearing up for a spare-tyre crisis as drivers and passengers become so fat that manufacturers are having to reconfigure their vehicles to accommodate them'.[29] Some may agree that, if corporations wanted to impact positively on these health and socio-economic issues of the day and consider the long term, then the right thing to do, excepting medical conditions, would be to leave 'the size of seats and grab handles' unchanged, encouraging those who maintain a healthy lifestyle with the 'privilege' of being able to drive a car.

From all national and international studies, it is becoming clear that poor diets are contributing more to health problems than any other cause. In an extensive and insightful evidence-based paper, Loren Cordain, professor and researcher in the Health and Exercise Science Department at Colorado State University, emphasises the importance of understanding basic human evolutionary processes in terms of the relationship between food and human biology.[30,31]

His main thesis is that 'the foods that humanity originally evolved to eat and those we now eat in modern civilization are in many cases significantly different – yet our basic underlying genetic inheritance remains basically the same it was before, and has only evolved slightly since. Thus many of the foods we now eat are discordant with our genetic inheritance.' The major shift occurred in the 'so-called "Agricultural Revolution" (primarily the domestication of animals, cereals, grains and legumes) in the Near East about 10,000 years ago and spread to northern Europe by about 5,000 years or so'. Throughout human evolution and 'virtually all the rest of the studied hunter-gatherer populations, cereal grains ("including wheat, corn, barley, rye, oats, millet and sorghum") were not consumed', and are therefore 'a relatively recent food for hominids and our physiologies are still adjusting and adapting to their presence'.

Interviewed by Dr Robert Crayon, a clinician, researcher and educator described as 'one of the top ten nutritionists in the country [United States]', Professor Cordain notes that according to the 'fossil record, early farmers, compared to their hunter-gatherer predecessors, had a characteristic reduction in stature, an increase in infant mortality, a reduction in lifespan, an increased incidence of infectious diseases, an increase in iron deficiency anemia, an increased incidence of osteomalacia, porotic hyperostosis and other bone mineral disorders in the number of dental caries and enamel defects'.[32]

While 'some populations have had c. 333 generations (since the Agricultural Revolution c. 10,000 years ago) to adapt to the new staple foods of agriculture, others have had only 1–3 (i.e. Inuit, Amerindian)', argues Professor Cordain. Moreover, 'when cereal grain calories reach 50% or more of the daily caloric intake,' he observes,' humans suffer severe health consequences, such as 'the severe pellagra epidemics of the late 19th century in America and the beri-beri scourges of southeast Asia to confirm this', with other research also implicating 'zinc deficiencies due to the effects of excessive cereal grain consumption in retarding skeletal growth'. The ratio of hunter-gatherer diets was about 35% plant and 65% animal foods. Although there are regional variations, with more balanced diets in some southern nations, the current African diet generally consists of cereals (50%–80%), oils and fats (20%) and animal products (7%–20%). Worldwide, as shown in Figure 1.7, the average diet consists largely of cereals (51%); oils, fats, sugars (19.5 %); milk, fish, eggs (13.5%); fruits, vegetables, pulses and nuts (8.2%); 5.3% of roots and tubers; and other (2.8%),[26] – quite different from the Palaeolithic diet that may be more in harmony with our genetic make-up.

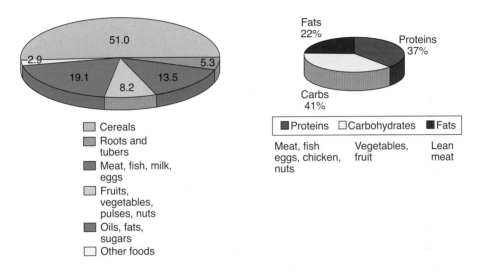

FIGURE 1.7 World average diet[33] versus Palaeolithic diet (adapted from Eaton SB 3rd, Konner MJ. Paleolithic nutrition revisited: a twelve-year retrospective on its nature and implications. *Eur J Clin Nutr*. 1997; **51**(4): 207–16)

Further, Professor Cordain remarks – and not without controversy from the medical establishment – that 'antinutritional components in raw cereal grains … wreak havoc with human health and well-being', in particular, 'the primary storage form of phosphorus in cereal grains – phytate' along with other antinutrients in cereal grains and legumes. 'Excessive consumption of whole grain unleavened bread (50%–60% of total calories) commonly results in rickets, retarded skeletal growth, and iron deficiency anaemia.' Further, 'antinutrients in wheat such as the wheat germ agglutinin and gliadin have adverse effects upon the gastrointestinal tract'. In terms of legumes (e.g. sprouts, beans), most 'are non-digestible and/or toxic to most mammals', containing a wide variety of antinutritional compounds that influence multiple tissues and systems, 'which normal cooking procedures do not always eliminate'.

Moreover, physician Tim Ferriss advises '[i]t is also clear that other autoimmune diseases such as rheumatoid arthritis, lupus, Sjögren's, multiple sclerosis and a host of other autoimmune conditions occur at much higher rates in celiac patients'. While cause and effect relationships are difficult to establish, it is noteworthy that wheat, a worldwide staple, represents that only known environmental trigger of any autoimmune disease. It is estimated that about 1 out of 133 people in the US and Europe have celiac disease.

Professor Cordain's and Dr Ferriss's findings and observations – along with those of other research scientists – find support in a 2007 study where a research team from Lund University, Sweden, 'noted a remarkable absence of cardiovascular disease and diabetes among the traditional population of Kitava, Trobriand Islands, Papua New Guinea, where modern agrarian-based food is unavailable'.[34] As Professor Cordain observes, 'before the advent of agriculture, during 2.5 million years of human evolution, our ancestors were consuming fruit, vegetables, nuts, lean meat and fish'.

In the first clinical study of its kind,[35] a research group in Sweden compared 14 patients 'who were advised to consume a Paleolithic diet for 3 months with 15 patients who followed the Mediterranean diet, which includes whole-grain cereals, low-fat dairy products, fruit, vegetables and refined fats' and is 'generally considered healthy'. All patients were pre-diabetic and most had overt diabetes type 2. All had been diagnosed with coronary heart disease. The group that followed the Mediterranean diet saw their blood sugar levels improve by 7%. But those who followed the Palaeolithic diet had a sugar improvement of 26%.

Dr Ferriss concludes that based on the fossil record our Neolithic ancestors lost an average of six inches in height versus our Palaeolithic ancestors because of the Neolithic diet of grains and legumes, mainly 'because of the action of antinutrients such as phytates combined with the gut damaging characteristics of lectins and protease inhibitors'.[31]

Malnutrition: 'the face of worldwide hunger'

While obesity is a major concern for high- and some low-income countries, malnutrition is largely a huge global challenge for poor nations, as shown in Figure 1.8. The World Hunger Education Service distinguishes between two types of malnutrition.[36] The first and most important, referred to when world hunger is discussed, is protein-energy malnutrition – the most lethal form of malnutrition/hunger is basically a lack of calories and protein – the lack of enough protein (from meat and other sources) and food that provides energy (measured in calories) which all of the basic food groups provide. The second type of malnutrition is micronutrient (vitamin and mineral) deficiency, but 'is not the type of malnutrition that is referred to when world hunger is discussed, though it is certainly very important'.

In 1996 the World Food Summit set a target 'adopted by the nations of the world … to halve the number of undernourished people by 2015 from their number in 1990–92'. This target was later adopted in the UN Millennium Development Goals,[6] along with the goal of reducing 'the proportion of people whose income is less than $1 a day'. In the early 1990s the estimated number of undernourished people in developing countries was 824 million. However, by 2009, 'the number had climbed to 1.02 billion people'. 'The present outcome indicates how marginal the efforts were in face of the real need.'[36]

Figure 1.8 provides an overview of the number of people who are undernourished in the world. According to Klaus von Grebmer, public relations manager of the International Food Policy Research Institute, the worst World Hunger Index (WHI) figures are in southern Asia and sub-Saharan Africa. 'In southern Asia this is primarily due to the low status of women in the field of nutrition and also education. In Africa, conflicts, poor governance and the high rates of AIDS explain the most important results.'[37]

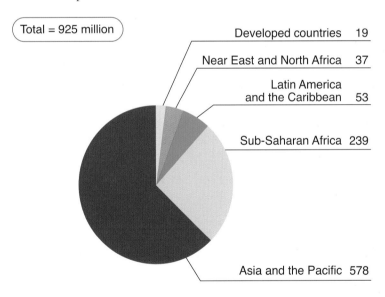

FIGURE 1.8 Number of hungry people in the world[36]

As '[i]t has life-long consequences for the health and capabilities of the people it affects', Bärbel Dieckmann, Welthungerhilfe's chairperson, highlights that '[m]alnutrition among infants under two years old represents one of the greatest challenges in the fight against hunger'. She pointed this out at the presentation of the 2010 Global Hunger Index, which in that year concentrated for the first time on the malnutrition of young children.[37]

Its most important conclusion is: the period between conception and the second year of life is crucial for development. If too little food, or the wrong kind of food, is available in these 1,000 days, the negative consequences of malnutrition are irreversible. Mothers who had a poor diet as children frequently give birth to underweight children. We have got to break this vicious circle of malnutrition by providing consistent advice and by rigorously promoting rural development.

The World Hunger Education Service provides compelling and distressing evidence in support of these concerns:

Children are the most visible victims of undernutrition. Children who are poorly nourished suffer up to 160 days of illness each year. Poor nutrition plays a role in at least half of the 10.9 million child deaths each year – five million deaths. Undernutrition magnifies the effect of every disease, including measles and malaria. The estimated proportions of deaths in which undernutrition is an underlying cause are roughly similar for diarrhea (56%), malaria (57%), pneumonia (52%), and measles (45%). Malnutrition can also be caused by diseases, such as the diseases that cause diarrhea, by reducing the body's ability to convert food into usable nutrients.[36]

Recalling Professor Cordain's[30] and Dr Ferriss's[31] observations discussed earlier, in developing countries we may be identifying some of the consequences of antinutrients and chronic undernourishment in Africa and Asia, most likely for the reasons that they and other researchers suggest, where 'about a third of all children under five years old are too small for their age, and therefore underdeveloped' and '[o]ver 90 percent of children who show signs of chronic undernourishment live in Africa and Asia'.[36]

The main causes of malnutrition relate to poverty, 'with an estimated 1,345 million people in developing countries who live on $1.25 a day or less'. Another major challenge results from harmful economic systems, where minority 'control over resources and income is based on military, political and economic power'. Ongoing conflicts and violence have also led to 'significant increase in refugee numbers'. It is well known that chronic undernutrition causes poor health, low levels of energy, and even mental impairment, leading 'to even greater poverty by reducing people's ability to work and learn, thus leading to even greater hunger'. Another factor contributing to malnutrition is climate change, by '[i]ncreasing drought, flooding, and changing climatic patterns requiring a shift in crops and farming practices that may not be easily accomplished'.[36]

Feeding the hungry is compounded by the present recession and price inflation with 'the current price index for a basket of essential, basic food items at its highest level since the FAO [Food and Agriculture Organization] began measuring prices in 1990'.[38] As examples, prices of wheat have increased by 84%, maize by 74%, sugar by 77%, and oils and fats by 57%. As a result, poor families around the globe commonly spend 40%–70% or more of their income on food. And, as mentioned previously, more than a quarter of the world's population still lives on $2 per day. Jason Corum, online communications manager at the US World Food Programme, in a 2011 report *World Food Prices Hit Record High*, calls for coordinated action 'to help poor people in developing countries cope with high food prices and stem future unrest and instability' and to 'invest in developing their agricultural sectors'.[38]

While these directions are crucial, particularly at this time of financial turbulence, the longer term may need re-evaluation in the light of Professor Cordain's[30] and others' research into the biological effects of certain foods.[31] If grains are basically harmful to the human body,[39] it appears imperative that alternative forms of nutritious foods – possibly through genetic modification of crops that are healthier for the human body and increasing the amount of low-fat meat in diets – are found to feed an increasingly hungry world in the twenty-first century. As mentioned previously, according to the FAO,[33] the average African diet is mainly cereal-based with very little protein, unlike Western diets which generally contain c. 20%–30% meat, fish, milk and eggs, but are also high in fats and sugars as well as carbohydrates. Both diets are clearly inadequate in terms of fruits, vegetables, pulses and nuts and help to explain malnutrition in poor countries and the disastrous rise of obesity and its unhealthy side effects in the richer nations. It would be impossible of course at this stage to consider a grain-free diet in developing nations as people depend on cereal grains as part of their staple diet. However, Western societies do have more food choices and grain-free diets could greatly reduce the rising levels of obesity.

As with other breakthroughs – 'especially the use of transgenic plants and animals for the production of new drugs and vaccines, xenotransplantation, and the like', promising cheaper, more universal healthcare, some of the answers for discovering more nourishing staple foods in the twenty-first century and improved living standards may lie with biotechnology,[40] along with decreasing child mortality rates, improved family planning and enhancing economic growth while optimising renewable energy.

Impact of rising costs on healthcare

In the previous sections we looked at the human costs related to obesity and malnutrition. As with all these serious issues affecting millions of lives, there is inevitably a pressure to reduce costs of healthcare, which have been growing exponentially since the early 1990s in most developed countries. Driven by junk food diets and a lack of exercise, in the United Kingdom the cost of obesity and diabetes to the NHS has been estimated at £9 billion per year – about 10% of the entire NHS budget, with the number of diabetes sufferers rising by 50% in just five years. Over three million adults and children now have the condition, after an increase of more than 117 000 in the 12 months to October 2011 alone.[41] Moreover, '[t]he number of elderly people admitted to hospital because they are dangerously fat has soared almost ten-fold in five years' in the United Kingdom.[42]

According to research carried out in North America by the Society of Actuaries, '[t]he total economic cost of an overweight and obese population in the U.S. and Canada approaches $300 billion per year, with 90 percent of the total – $270 billion – attributed to the U.S.'[43]

In the study, the Society of Actuaries also divided the $300 billion finding into specific causes of economic costs. It is likely that these figures reflect proportionality in other countries.

- Total cost of excess medical care caused by overweight and obesity: $127 billion.
- Economic loss of productivity caused by excess mortality: $49 billion.
- Economic loss of productivity caused by disability for active workers: $43 billion.
- Economic loss of productivity caused by overweight or obesity for totally disabled workers: $72 billion.

In another study it was estimated that obesity costs US businesses approximately $73 billion per year, which 'stems primarily from excess medical cost along with lost workplace productivity'.[44] In addition, the US spends more than $150 billion annually on healthcare linked to obesity, and according to Risa Lavizzo-Mourey, president and chief executive officer of the Robert Wood Johnson Foundation, '[o]besity is the driver of so many chronic conditions – heart disease, diabetes, cancer – that generate the exorbitant costs that are crushing our health-care system … The biggest driver of these excess costs are prescription drugs.' And, '[a]mong the normal-weight population, prescription drug costs average about $700 a year, but among those who are obese the cost rises to about $1,300 a year, an 80 percent increase'.[45]

In 2011 more than two-thirds of the UK NHS budget, which has risen sharply in the last 20 years (about £29 billion in 1994 to over £100 billion currently),[46] is being spent on chronic care. These figures will most likely increase substantially in the coming years, triggering reduced income streams for medical education and possible erosion of 'the clinical environment',[47] including research funding.[48] Moreover, decreasing family size in most developed countries – European and North American – will make affordability of health and social care more difficult, as projected in the dependency ratio, 'calculated by dividing the number of people of working age by the number of people of retirement age'. In the United Kingdom, for example, it is estimated that the current ratio is 3:1 (working for each retired individual), decreasing to 2:1 by 2041.[49]

Globally, as shown in Figure 1.9, 'inequality in healthcare spending is large' with 'countries in the highest quintile (20%)' spending 'more than 16 times the amount spent by the lowest quintile'.[50] 'National Geographic has published an infographic that uses OECD Health Data 2009 and information from the Organisation for Economic Co-operation and Development to show relationships between health care spending per person (on the left [Figure 1.9]) and the average life expectancy at birth (on the right). The thickness of the line indicates the average number of doctor visits a year. ... Ideally, most lines (should be) going up-and-to-the-right, meaning a low cost of health-care, but a high life expectancy.' Unfortunately, according to Randall Hand, a visualisation scientist working for a US federal research lab, 'that bright orange line diving drastically downward is the US, having the highest health care spending of all shown nations, and a slightly lower than average life expectancy'.[51]

As Figure 1.9 indicates, there is not necessarily a correlation between healthcare spending and life expectancy. Japan spends less than most countries but has the world's best life expectancy for both males and females. Japanese citizens also have the most visits to doctors. In light of the data, there can be little doubt that healthy diet and lifestyle contribute considerably to a longer life.

Although the United States spends more than any other country on health, it ranks 27th in terms of life expectancy, at about the same level as Cuba, where per capita spending is only about US$200 per person.

In a *New Economist* Buttonwood blog,[52] 'named after the 1792 agreement that regulated the informal brokerage conducted under a buttonwood tree on Wall Street', the columnist cites a recent paper in the *International Journal of Epidemiology*, 'Trends in European life expectancy: a salutary view',[53] which 'points to the continuing improvement in European longevity. Among the striking findings are the declines in longevity in ex-Soviet Union states like Latvia and Lithuania, alongside the better-known deterioration in Russia.' Further, the anonymous blogger notes: 'It also seems remarkable that life expectancy in the US is now on a par with the worst countries in western Europe (Portugal for men and, surprisingly, Denmark for women). Life expectancy for US women has been increasing very slowly relative to Europe.' In contrast,

> [as] the author of the paper, David Leon, points out, much of Europe has improved longevity at a similar rate, despite differences in health systems. Much seems to be down to a decline in cardiovascular disease mortality which may in turn be linked to the decline in smoking rates (Denmark was slower to give up, apparently). This parallelism may be a product of the sort of

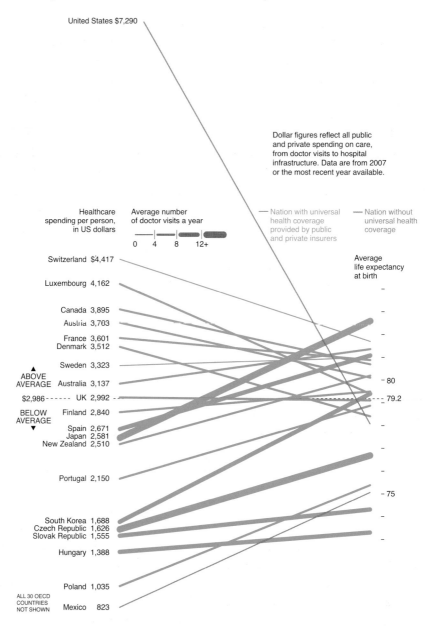

FIGURE 1.9 'Health care spending: large differences, unequal results'[51]

diffusion of knowledge and ideas that occurs in a connected world ... whereby improvements in public health or medical treatment and personal behaviours all make small but incremental contributions whose net effect is to reduce mortality. This reinforces the idea that primary care (public health, better personal habits) gets more bang for the buck than the expensive technological approach often used in the US.

Professor Leon[53] adds in his paper that 'it has been argued in the USA that the positive effects of smoking decline may be overwhelmed by the negative effects of increasing obesity. But that also raises the question of why Europeans, who have as much access to fast food as Americans, haven't got as fat.'

Comparing health metrics across seven countries, a Commonwealth Fund study[54] looked at five key dimensions: quality; access; efficiency; equity; and long, healthy and productive lives (*see* Figure 1.10). In 2010, as in 2004, 2006 and 2007, 'the United States ranked last when compared to Britain, Canada, Germany, Netherlands, Australia and New Zealand'. Health spending was US$7290 per person in the United States, more than double that of any other country in the survey and that excluded 46 million who were not insured, leading Jeffrey Flier, dean of Harvard Medical School, to comment that 'the US health-care system suffers from problems of cost, access and quality and needs major reform'. The main reasons, he points out, are that '[t]ax policy drives employment-based insurance; this begets overinsurance and drives costs upward while creating inequities for the unemployed and self-employed'. In addition, 'a regulatory morass limits innovation. And deep flaws in Medicare and Medicaid drive spending without optimising care.'[55]

As shown in Figure 1.10, using a 7-point rating scale (where 1 = excellent), there is no correlation between expenditures and the quality metrics. Improvements are needed in all countries.[54]

As already mentioned, there are similar issues in the other countries studied, although certainly not as severe as in the United States. New Zealand spent the least, at US$2454, but New Zealand is first in terms of quality of care, and 'Canada and the U.S. rank sixth and seventh overall, respectively', having spent more than the other five countries.

Three of the countries – Canada, the Netherlands and the United Kingdom – have a poor rating for 'patient-centred care', which has been a pivotal shift, at least philosophically, in the last decade or so. One conclusion of this data is that 'many patients do not get the degree of involvement they desire … and that patients were less likely than others to be given a self-management plan for chronic conditions, or advice on preventing ill health'.[49] Poor physician–patient communication and 'professionals as authorities' versus 'professionals as partners', a theme discussed in later chapters of this book, may also contribute to the ratings.

'The most notable way the U.S. differs from other countries is the absence of universal health insurance coverage.' However, '[h]ealth reform legislation recently signed into law by President Barack Obama should begin to improve the affordability of insurance and access to care when fully implemented in 2014'.[54] Somewhat surprisingly, Germany, which is well known for its efficiency in manufacturing, does rather poorly in terms of 'effective care', 'coordinated care' and, indeed, 'efficiency'.

Exhibit ES-1. Overall Ranking

Country Rankings	
	1.00–2.33
	2.34–4.66
	4.67–7.00

	AUS	CAN	GER	NETH	NZ	UK	US
OVERALL RANKING (2010)	3	6	4	1	5	2	7
Quality care	4	7	5	2	1	3	6
Effective care	2	7	6	3	5	1	4
Safe care	6	5	3	1	4	2	7
Co-ordinated care	4	5	7	2	1	3	6
Patient-centred care	2	5	3	6	1	7	4
Access	6.5	5	3	1	4	2	6.5
Cost-related problem	6	3.5	3.5	2	5	1	7
Timeliness of care	6	7	2	1	3	4	5
Efficiency	2	6	5	3	4	1	7
Equity	4	5	3	1	6	2	7
Long, healthy, productive lives	1	2	3	4	5	6	7
Health expenditures/capita, 2007	$3,357	$3,895	$3,588	$3,837*	$2,454	$2,992	$7,290

Note: *Estimate. Expenditures shown in $US PPP (purchasing power parity).
Source: Calculated by The Commonwealth Fund based on 2007 International Health Policy Survey; 2008 International Health Policy Survey of Sicker Adults; 2009 International Health Policy Survey of Primary Care Physicians; Commonwealth Fund Commission on a High Performance Health System National Scorecard; and Organization for Economic Cooperation and Development, OECD Health Data, 2009 (Paris: OECD, Nov. 2009).

FIGURE 1.10 Commonwealth Fund study: overall country rankings[54]

As Figures 1.11 and 1.12 illustrate, and as previously mentioned, average spending on health and total expenditures on health as a percentage of gross domestic product also varied markedly across these seven countries, with Australia, the United Kingdom and New Zealand in the lower tier for both and the United States at the top, followed by Germany and Canada.[45]

Although it is relatively easy to explain why healthcare costs are low in some countries, it becomes more difficult to justify very high expenditures, such as those in Canada and the United States. This discussion, although beyond the scope of this book, is reviewed briefly further in Chapter 8. Reasons for this variance may come down to, as Dean Flier at Harvard has mentioned,[55] not only

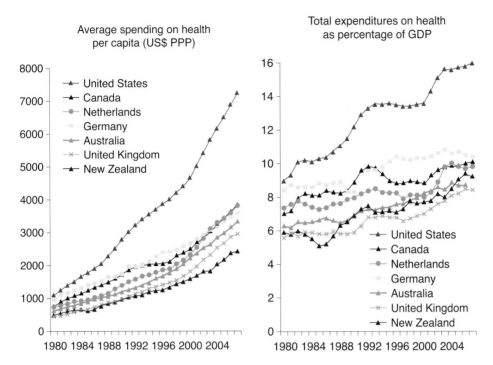

Average spending on health
per capita (US$ PPP)

Total expenditures on health
as percentage of GDP

- United States
- Canada
- Netherlands
- Germany
- Australia
- United Kingdom
- New Zealand

FIGURE 1.11 Average spending on health per capita (US$ purchasing power parity)

FIGURE 1.12 Total expenditure on health as percentage of gross domestic product

tax policy and employment-based insurance but also poor lifestyle choices (e.g. obesity and diabetes, cardiovascular problems, cancers), cost of technological interventions, imbalance in specialist and general practitioner ratios and public demand for instant action. As one senior member of the medical profession has pointed out: 'Americans won't wait. Putting off breast surgery or heart surgery for months does not fly in this country. We are still a capitalistic society and health care is part of it. ... Many of the European countries view health care as a right and not a privilege – I happen to agree – but many in America do not believe that and therefore having a national health plan is not in the works.' Arguably, there has also been a reluctance by governments to tackle large corporations (e.g. regarding smoking, pharmaceuticals, air pollution and so forth).

Considering expenditures on professional health education alone presents many imbalances across the world. *The Lancet* Commission reports that '[w]orldwide there are 2420 medical schools, 467 schools or departments of public health, and an indeterminate number of postsecondary nursing educational institutions'.[56] These 'train about 1 million new doctors, nurses, midwives, and public health professionals every year'. Further, the commissioners emphasise that '[s]evere institutional shortages are exacerbated by maldistribution, both between and within countries. Four countries (China, India, Brazil, and USA) each have more than 150 medical schools, whereas 36 countries have no medical schools at all. Twenty-six countries in sub-Saharan Africa have one or no medical schools. … In view of these imbalances [the fact that] medical school numbers do not align well with either country population size or national burden of disease is not surprising.'

Another serious issue relates to '[t]he total global expenditure for health professional education'. Worldwide, the cost of health professional education 'is about US$100 billion per year, again with great disparities between countries'. Alarmingly, the Commission underscores that '[t]his amount is less than 2% of health expenditures worldwide, which is pitifully modest for a labour-intensive and talent-driven industry'. A comparative case in point indicates that in the United States even the highest expenditure on professional education (about $55 billion) 'for all activities by medical schools is barely 2% of the $2.5 trillion spent in 2009'. These figures are disappointing when compared with other expenditures in the United States, as noted in *The Lancet* report – US$34 billion spent on 'yoga, massage, meditation and natural products and $23 billion, on dietary and vitamin supplements'.[56]

In terms of the cost per graduate, the Commission estimates that the average cost is '$113 000 for medical students and $46 000 for nurses, with unit costs highest in North America and lowest in China'. Moreover, *The Lancet* Commission concludes that '[s]tewardship, accreditation, and learning systems are weak and unevenly practised around the world'. The Commission's 'analysis has shown the scarcity of information and research about health professional education' and, although 'many educational institutions in all regions have launched innovative initiatives, little robust evidence is available about the effectiveness of such reforms'.

Given the depth of the recession, it is unlikely that most governments (other than China and perhaps other 'growth economies' such as Brazil, Russia and India – the BRIC economies) will have the means to increase funding for professional education. One option for governments might be to identify areas of high, but possibly less impactful, expenditures and to re-route funding to professional education, which, as has been argued, requires radical change. Another choice may be to secure private investments in professional education, but, according to *The Lancet* Commission, this increasing reliance 'generates concern about quality and social purpose'. Similar to uncoordinated and unregulated expansion of medical schools in the United States in the latter half of the nineteenth century, '[d]riven by global workforce shortages and growing market demand for health services, a large increase in unplanned and unregulated medical schools could generate the very same type of low-quality proprietary schools that Flexner visited, criticised and successfully closed'.

Accreditation is also an issue. 'China has about 1 million village doctors and India has about 1 million rural medical practitioners who are not graduates of accredited schools.'[56] These 2 million practitioners, as well as many others in most countries, 'are not graduates of accredited schools'.[56] *The Lancet* Commission advocates the introduction of social accountability – 'directing education, research and service activities towards addressing the priority health concerns of the community' – into accreditation. Pursuing this direction could be 'instrumental in the production of a professional workforce that is well aligned with societal health goals, including equity, quality, and efficiency'.[56]

Unsurprisingly, increased demand for healthcare services and decreased levels of funding have led to a dilemma in many countries. One of the direct consequences has been the time that a patient can be seen by a qualified professional. For example, in the United Kingdom 'the number of people who have had to wait for more than six months for treatment has increased by 56%, and the number waiting more than four hours in Accident & Emergency has doubled in the past year, despite a fall in attendance.'[57] This situation has caused frustration and in some cases led to people taking desperate measures, as outlined in the following extract relating to a 41-year-old man in British Columbia, Canada.

> He entered the emergency room at 8 p.m. complaining of symptoms resembling a heart attack. After not being attended to for 45 minutes, he left the emergency department and returned later that night at 11 p.m. At this point he began to become unruly and threatened to drive his vehicle through the emergency room doors if he did not receive medical attention. He was then told by the staff to calm down or they would have to contact the police. He was not seen by a physician so he left the emergency room untreated for a second time that night. At this point he followed through with his promise by driving his 1987 Chevy Blazer through the ER double doors and into its hallway. Luckily, nobody within the ER department was injured. Police officers arrived a short while later and arrested the man who was still behind the wheel of his vehicle. Even after all the events that unfolded, it is still unclear if he was seen by a doctor.[58]

In the United States things are not much different – maybe worse – as 'both data and anecdotes show that the American people are already waiting as long or longer than patients living with universal health-care systems'.[59]

> Take Susan M., a 54-year-old human resources executive in New York City. She faithfully makes an appointment for a mammogram every April, knowing the wait will be at least six weeks. She went in for her routine screening at the end of May, then had another because the first wasn't clear. That second X-ray showed an abnormality, and the doctor wanted to perform a needle biopsy, an outpatient procedure. His first available date: mid-August. 'I completely

freaked out,' Susan says. 'I couldn't imagine spending the summer with this hanging over my head.' After many calls to five different facilities, she found a clinic that agreed to read her existing mammograms on June 25 and promised to schedule a follow-up MRI and biopsy if needed within 10 days. A full month had passed since the first suspicious X-rays. Ultimately, she was told the abnormality was nothing to worry about, but she should have another mammogram in six months. Taking no chances, she made an appointment on the spot. 'The system is clearly broken,' she laments.

One observer comments that '[a]ll this time spent "queuing," as other nations call it, stems from too much demand and too little supply. Only one-third of U.S. doctors are general practitioners, compared with half in most European countries. On top of that, only 40% of U.S. doctors have arrangements for after-hours care, vs. 75% in the rest of the industrialized world. Consequently, some 26% of U.S. adults in one survey went to an emergency room in the past two years because they couldn't get in to see their regular doctor, a significantly higher rate than in other countries.'[59]

Further, unlike some other countries that have national health systems, it is difficult to draw comparisons, as in the United States '[t]here is no systemised collection of data on wait times. However, a 2005 survey by the Commonwealth Fund of sick adults in six nations found that only 47% of U.S. patients could get a same- or next-day appointment for a medical problem, worse than every other country except Canada.'

According to *BusinessWeek*, '[f]ew solutions have been proposed … in part, say policy experts, because the problem is rarely acknowledged'. However, increasingly, 'the market is beginning to address the issue with the rise of walk-in medical clinics…. These retail clinics promise rapid care for minor medical problems, usually getting patients in and out in 30 minutes.' The slogan for one of these 'Minute Clinics says it all: You're sick. We're quick.'[59]

Australian data are better than those in other countries with waiting for general surgery about 36 days and emergency waiting times averaging just 24 minutes. There are still challenges, as noted by Australian Medical Association former national president Dr Andrew Pesce, who considered that 'it is disappointing there has been no major improvement despite additional federal funding' and that 'the only way hospital performance will improve is when there is targeted funding for extra beds to allow patients to be treated in a timely way, because the emergency department is blocked up with patients who are spending time there when they should actually be admitted to the hospital proper'.[60]

As may be the case in other countries, reluctance in the United States to become involved in change and improvements in healthcare is pervasive – perhaps becoming less so when the money runs out. By the end of 2010 only one state had worked with the Federal Government on its healthcare reforms and proactively started 'instituting those changes in its legislation to re-empower the doctors and nurses and other health professionals'.[59] Further, paralleling major themes from several international reports on medical education,[56] Dr Pesce reminded his audience about the importance of coming up 'with local solutions, utilising the local workforce and the local facilities and the local infrastructure to get the best outcomes for our patients'.[60]

Nor are the problems confined to doctors. Professor DJ Thomas, a retired UK consultant neurologist, notes that '[m]edical contemporaries, having observed changes over the past 40 years, dread the thought of being admitted to hospital at the mercy of nursing staff with poor caring skills'.[62] He links the decline in care 'to the obsession that all nurses must work for a degree. So in their formative early years nurses spend less time in a compassionate workplace and more in a detached lecture room', as do, arguably, most future healthcare professionals.

Rejecting this view, and writing in the same newspaper 'Letter to the Editor'[62] section of *The Times*, a nursing student who quit her training points out that '[w]ard staff levels operate at a minimum in most departments, meaning student nurses cannot learn these skills simply because the staff do not have time to teach them'. She reflects that she spent 2 years undergoing nurse training and the majority of time on the wards was spent doing basic yet important tasks that did not require supervision, such as taking temperatures and running up and down stairs to collect prescriptions. She mentions further that as a '[s]upernumery student' she 'was not missed when off the ward' and like many of her colleagues had 'no other option but to work part time alongside their 37-plus hours a week on the wards'. She concludes that '[i]t's almost impossible to learn effectively when exhausted but students need to pay their bills and so, like a large percentage of my cohort, I left'.

'Under the old system,' exclaims Camilla Cavendish, a British columnist and leader writer for *The Times*,[63] 'student nurses were paid as part of the ward team and were valuable to that team, so got good supervised experience'. Another serious issue that she mentions relates to the removal of student nurses from ward teams, thereby creating a hole in the workforce that was filled by a new cohort of people called healthcare assistants, who are 'lower paid auxiliaries who are supposed to be supervised by a registered nurse but at chaotic times are not'. The healthcare assistants 'have almost no training … [and] do non-medical tasks such as feeding and washing. … In other words,' Cavendish admonishes, 'we have delegated the hands-on care that patients value to the lowest-paid untrained people, some of whom find it hard to communicate well in English.' Her final comment is that 'to give someone a bed bath with dignity, to stop them getting bedsores, to persuade them to eat … can be as important to recovery as medicine. Yet we increasingly delegate it to 300,000 healthcare assistants who are not only untrained but also unregulated.' This lack of patient support is especially stress-ful and harmful for elderly patients, many of whom, according to Care Quality Commission inspections undertaken of NHS wards, 'are routinely left without anything to drink for hours, with some so dehydrated they are put on drips'.[64]

While noting this troubling state of affairs, Cavendish has also seen 'exemplary nursing care', usually from those who work in places 'with superb management, where teamwork is valued, standards are high and accountability is clear'. The status quo 'that has moved too many nurses away from patient care' is not toler-able, as admitted by Peter Carter, head of the Royal College of Nursing. The issue has become so intense in the United Kingdom that a leading NHS hospital trust has decided to set up its own nurse training scheme based on the premise that some nursing degrees are too academic and are neglecting 'attitudes and behaviour'. According to Kerry Jones, dean of the trust's faculty of education: '[i]t's about compassion, holding a patient's hand if they need it – for people to get well you have to get the fundamentals right'.[65] The question that remains – a question that Jones asks too – if the training scheme is a success is 'will other parts of the health service follow'?

Improving health literacy

Poor health literacy, generally attributed to racial and ethnic disparities, contribut-ing 'to the vicious circle of poor health from one generation to the next',[49] remains a serious cause for concern for most nations. Research has shown that patients with poor health literacy are 'at greatest risk of misunderstanding their diagnoses, medications and instructions on how to take care of their medical problems'. In the United States, for example, it is estimated that about '75 million English-speaking adults have limited health literacy', leading to 'higher risk of death and more emergency room visits and hospitalizations'.[66]

In an informative presentation by the Molina HealthCare and California Academy of Family Physicians, entitled *I Hear You Talking, But I Don't Understand You!' Medical jargon and clear communication*,[67] the speaker makes the point that '[j]argon is a language of familiarity. It can be a useful tool when everyone has a common understanding of the terms at hand – it is verbal shorthand. The problems arise when physicians let jargon creep into their everyday communica-tion with patients. This is when physician language can separate, insulate and intimidate. Good communication is the result of the use of common terms that are clearly understood by both parties.'

In terms of a national response, the US National Action Plan to Improve Health Literacy must be seen as a step in the right direction and possibly worthy of consideration by other nations. The plan calls for improving the 'jargon-filled

language, dense writing, and complex explanations that often fill patient han
outs, medical forms, health web sites and recommendations to the public'.[68]

It is for some of these reasons that governments, pressed for funds, are
seeking alternatives to how people are currently accessing healthcare. There
is a gradual move, in the main, from costly hospital care to localised primary
care[69] and community-based teams of professionals while insisting that the individual increasingly take personal responsibility for his or her own well-being. As
Professor Lord Ara Darzi, chair for the Institute of Global Health Innovation at
the UK Imperial College,[70] points out, the likelihood of localising some surgery is
already being supported through the separation of elective and emergency surgery
and the introduction of Diagnostic Treatment Centres and Independent Surgical
Treatment Centres. He also sees surgical possibilities (e.g. from endoscopies to
hernia repairs, cataracts, varicose vein treatments) in community hospitals, health
centres and primary care, such as large general practitioner practices. One recent
study confirmed that 'up to 80% of patients previously referred to hospital for
routine surgical procedures can be dealt with using purpose designed facilities
in a former cottage hospital'.[71]

While we need, unfortunately, to acknowledge that many nations still have
pre-industrial or no healthcare, in developed countries there is a shift, as previously discussed, from 'industrial age care' – with its Taylorian principles of
hierarchy, vertical management and low responsiveness – to information age care
that, it is expected, will place greater value on human dignity, shared decision-
making, choice and access to social care supports (*see* Figure 1.13).[72]

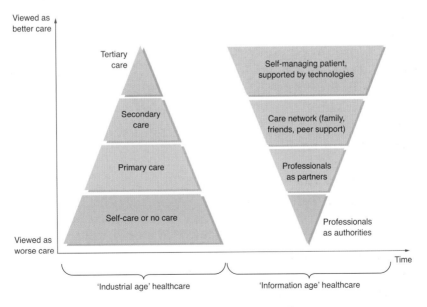

FIGURE 1.13 Industrial versus information age healthcare[73]

As already mentioned, in terms of philosophical assumptions underpinning healthcare, the longer-term view is that there will be a shift from 'a curative model based on the management and elimination of disease to a new archetype emphasising health capital', coupled with new ways of measuring health.[74] In this scenario, it is argued the more consideration will need to be ascribed by providers to the interplay between physical health, mental health and holistic health – paying increasing attention to genetic, socio-economic, psychological and biological factors (*see* Figure 1.14). These changes will strongly impact on how medical and social care will be provided, raising a potentially serious social concern about the health carer to pensioner ratio in various communities which, according to a 2009 Organisation for Economic Co-operation and Development (OECD) report,[75] is inadequate in many countries.

The transition to community care will also have an impact on the structure and content of health profession curricula at both undergraduate and postgraduate levels. For example, more emphasis will be required on balancing technical and adaptive skills (*see* Chapter 3 for further discussion), in particular how to optimise 'personal' care through effective communication and empathy and discussing ways of promoting self-care and engaging care networks.

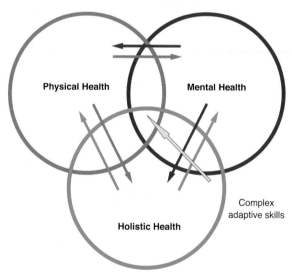

FIGURE 1.14 Whole-person integrated curricula[76]

Global health: 'putting families and communities at the hub'

A quick glance at population-per-doctor ratios, along with other 'vital statistics' across the globe,[77] paints a disturbing picture, with ratios in Africa of 25 000:1 in at least four countries, 33 500:1 in four countries, 50 000:1 in two countries and 20 000:1 in four countries. In India the patient-to-doctor ratio is about 1722:1, while in China it stands at about 950:1, similar to most South American countries. Japan, with the highest life expectancy, sits at about 500:1.

According to *The World Health Report 2006*,[11] worldwide there are approximately 1.3 billion people without healthcare, and there is a global shortfall of about 4.3 million healthcare workers. Most affected by these figures are of course the growing number of those who are starving in the world, living in many cases on less than US$1 per day.[6]

This shortage – doctors, nurses, midwives – has caused a crisis in at least 57 countries. In a cautiously optimistic paper, Dayrit, Dolea and Dreesch[78] report that 'world-wide ... health worker to population density fell below a critical threshold of 2.3 per 1,000 population. This means that below this critical threshold, a country could not provide the basic health services to its population, defined here as 80% immunisation coverage and 80% skilled birth attendance at delivery. Of the 57 countries, 36 are located in Africa.'

Addressing the crises has included effective planning with other stakeholders (e.g. health, education, finance), underpinned 'by developing a strong knowledge base', sustaining investments and 'the building of a critical mass of leaders and managers to guide the process'. While outcomes of these interventions have been variable, there have been notable successes, with 45 out of 57 (79%) of the countries developing human resources for health plans and 32 (71%) adopting an implementation budget and with 51 (89%) now having a human resources for health department in the ministry of health. Strategic plans generally focused on pre- and in-service education, education targets (number of health workers to be trained), career development, and incentives (e.g. payment, housing, transport). Reviewing health performance evaluation data of eight countries (Malawi, Peru, Ethiopia, Brazil, Thailand, the Philippines, Zambia and Mali), Dr Dayrit and others identified many examples of progress from raising densities of health worker to population in Malawi, to developing the concept of Family Health Teams in Peru, and to shifting from 'specialised, urban-centre, hospital-based medical care' to family health teams in Brazil. Keys to future successes for all nations appear to reside with 'political will, adequate investments and effective management over the long term'.

The developed world ratios pale in comparison with the low-income countries, with both France and Germany at 300:1; the United States, 390:1; Canada, 470:1; and Britain at 440:1.[11] The demographic, health and educational data in Figure 1.15 are indicative of the huge inequities that exist across the globe and the enormous challenges that face this and future generations. Considering the global village of 100 people, only one person has a university degree and only one person has a computer.

If you could fit the entire population of the world into a village consisting of 100 people, maintaining the proportions of all the people living on Earth, that village would consist of:

57 Asians

21 Europeans

14 Americans (North, Central and South)

8 Africans

52 women and 48 men

80 people who live in poverty

70 illiterate people

50 people suffering from hunger and malnutrition

1 person with a university degree

1 person with a computer

FIGURE 1.15 The global community: 'putting things in perspective'[79]

As previously noted, annual government expenditures on healthcare range from US$20 per person[50] to over US$7000.[51] The gap in life expectancy between developed and some developing countries is now about 40 years, with a number of countries evidencing 'high maternal, infant and under-five mortality', indicating 'lack of access to basic services such as clean water and sanitation, immunisations and proper nutrition'. While 'remarkable strides have been made to improve health, combat disease and lengthen life spans … translation of Primary HC [healthcare] values – social justice and the right to better health for all, participation and solidarity – has been uneven across the world with many people, including those in developed countries, dissatisfied with current health systems. Along with escalating costs, rather than improving their response capacity and anticipating new challenges, health systems seem to be drifting from one short-term priority to another, increasingly fragmented and without a clear sense of direction.' Based on cost-benefit analyses, those countries 'where health care is organised around the tenets of primary care produce a higher level of health for the same investment.'[56]

According to the World Health Organization, as mentioned before, reorientation of healthcare involves increasingly shifting from biomedical intervention to prevention and calls for a return to primary healthcare – and 'to bring balance back to health care and put families and communities at the hub of the health system'.[80] In addition, WHO director-general Margaret Chan, writing in an editorial for *The Lancet*, stresses that '[a]bove all, primary health care offer(s) a way to organise the full range of health care, from households to hospitals, with prevention equally important as cure, and with resources invested rationally in the different levels of care'.[80]

Tackling inequalities, WHO proposes that countries adopt four primary health care principles.

1. *Universal coverage*: ensuring that all people have access to healthcare.
2. *People-centred services*: with 'delivery points embedded in communities'.
3. *Healthy public policies*: ensuring that 'health in all policies' approach is integrated broadly throughout governments (e.g. trade, environment, education).
4. *Leadership*: requiring the capacity to 'negotiate and steer' and 'knowledge of what works', ensuring all stakeholders (including 'vulnerable groups') have a voice.[56]

Supporting the WHO proposals, *The Lancet* commissioners contend that:

> [p]rimary health-care training should be seamlessly integrated into the overall health system, including the academic system. Professional education has to reinforce the primary function of assuring access to high quality services for a defined population through proactive strategies, favouring continuity of care, guaranteeing an explicit set of entitlements [discussed further in Chapter 6], and assuring universal; social protection in health. The challenge for academic systems is to provide a more balanced environment for the education of professionals through engagement with local communities, to proactively address population-based prevention, anticipate future health threats, and to lead in the overall design and management of the health system.[56]

Scientific megatrends in healthcare and information technology

Scientific megatrends[81] are making their presence felt daily, involving such key areas as genomics with the capacity to predict diseases to come later in life; vaccines that may treat not only infections but also many chronic diseases 'from coronary artery disease to multiple sclerosis to cancer', thereby becoming 'the cornerstone of much of medicine, especially preventive medicine'. Advances are also taking place in radiology 'in molecular imaging with emphasis on functional or physiological imaging rather than atomic imaging' with the ability to uncover 'the process of disease rather than the location or shape of disease'. Simulators for operating room practice and robotic surgery including telesurgery are also becoming increasingly important. Undoubtedly, many advances will lead to new diagnostic capabilities and treatments, use of expert systems, and miniaturisation of diagnostic and treatments tools. On the downside, development costs are very high and the cost of treatment may become a major barrier for many people.

'While IT [information technology] has changed the relationships between learners and teacher', *The Lancet* commissioners emphasise, 'so too is it rapidly transforming the relationships between health professionals and the people they serve – be it individual patients or entire communities … advanced information technology is important not only for more efficient education of health professionals; its existence also demands a change in expected competencies. … Put simply,' the report authors affirm,

> the education of health professionals in the 21st century must focus less on memorising and transmitting facts and more on promotion of the reasoning and communication skills that will enable the professional to be an effective partner, facilitator, adviser and advocate.[56]

These skills and roles could increasingly be put to the test in transnational projects that use networked technology and telemedicine in supporting health-care workers and patients across the globe, particularly in developing countries, on a remote basis, providing capacity for telediagnostics, medical guidance, intensive care and training. As the authors of *Health Professionals for a New Century*[56] note:

> In poor countries, a major constraint is the scarcity of qualified teachers who are essential for training the next generation of professionals, including the training of basic health workers. Indeed, to achieve an expansion of the workforce in poor countries without ramping up faculty teaching resources is difficult. Of the options that deserve exploration is the short-term placement of graduates from rich countries seeking opportunities to contribute in other countries that are severely deficient in faculty. Such activities, however, should be part of a broader strategy for capacity strengthening in poor countries. IT can play a major part in this regard through the types of open educational resources.

The Lancet commissioners justifiably praise the OpenCourseWare (OCW) initiative, started in 2001, at the Massachusetts Institute of Technology, providing 'digitised material offered freely and openly for educators, students, and self-learners to use and re-use for teaching, learning and research'. The scheme has allowed 'many universities to share online their syllabi, lectures, assignments, and examinations free for others to download, modify and use'. Remarkably, '[b]y 2009, OCW had more than 200 member universities, with more than 6,200 courses freely online attracting more that 2 million visits per month'. OCW members include 'leading universities in the USA, China, Japan, Spain, Latin America, Korea, Turkey, and Vietnam, and regional networks adapted to local languages have been built in Latin America, China and Japan'. It is worth mentioning that 'Johns Hopkins University Bloomberg School of Public Health started its OCW project in 2005, and is now offering 60 graduate courses on line with an average of 40,000 visits per month' and that 'Tufts University now offers more than half its medical courses online'.[56]

There can be no doubt that 'OCW has the potential to transform health professional education through provision of free and open access to all interested learners worldwide, including developing countries that are severely limited by educational resources'. Another key benefit of OCW is that content quality can be continuously and globally improved 'through sharing of materials for feedback'.

Breaking down inter/trans-professional barriers

Globally, interprofessional and transdisciplinary teamworking has a long history. Midwives were mentioned in the Old Testament, and it was a recognised profession in ancient Egypt and Graeco-Roman times. While midwives were used in the early eighteenth century, surgeons largely replaced midwives in the early nineteenth century. Nursing is relatively speaking a newer profession, with both men and women engaged in nursing in seventeenth-century Europe often as a form of punishment. The roots of the profession as we know it were laid in the 1850s, with Florence Nightingale and her nurses treating the wounded during the Crimean War.[82] Largely because of Nightingale's efforts, '[t]he first nursing education programme began in London in 1859, as 2-year hospital-based training that soon spread quickly in the UK, the USA, Germany and Scandinavian countries'. The 'Goldman Report' in 1923 underscored nursing as a specialised field, calling 'for university-based schools of nursing, citing the inadequacies of existing educational facilities for training skilled nurses'. It is also noteworthy that the Commission on education of health professionals for the twenty-first century conclude that the 'report put nursing on the same trajectory as medicine and public health in the USA, albeit a little later in time'.[56]

However, today, while professionals – social workers, nurses, therapists, doctors, counsellors and so forth – work together in treating patients with non-communicable and infectious diseases as well as involvement in the prevention and control of injuries, by and large, they develop their knowledge and skills separately. This situation has come about despite having to treat patients 'from home to hospital to rehabilitation facilities' or requiring 'command and control teams involving surveillance, immunisation, containment, treatment, and interventions'.

Unlike the earlier part of the twentieth century, as Victor Yanchick, former chair of the Council of Deans of the American Association of Colleges of Pharmacy, points out, there are 'now virtually dozens of trained individuals' who have responsibility for patient care. However, 'for the most part each of these individuals is educated separately, in a closed system, without the opportunity to meaningfully interact with others until they complete their education'.[83]

The importance of the need to learn to collaborate better interprofessionally was brought to a head in London, in 2000, with the death of an 8-year-old Ivorian girl, Victoria Adjo Climbié. The young girl had been murdered by her guardians, leading to a public inquiry,[84] which produced major changes in child protection. The case revealed the poor communication and coordination among health and social care agencies, including the police, and led to the introduction of interprofessional learning programmes in a number of healthcare programmes.

In terms of healthcare, hallmarks of good patient care are leadership and collaboration, both of which are optimally learned and practised through regular, frequent and informal professional interactions in clinical and non-clinical environments at all levels and not just after graduation. Interprofessional educators define interprofessional education as '[o]ccasions when two or more professions learn with, from and about each other to improve collaboration and quality of care'.[85] With the aim of achieving the new professionalism, international practice networks call on 'accreditation bodies to include competencies in interprofessional education and collaborative practice within their validation, qualification, and revalidation requirements'.[86]

For example, in the early years of the last decade it became apparent that more needed to be done to encourage teamwork in the NHS.[87,88] This realisation was partly triggered by reports from service failures, and evidence that effective teamworking is positively related to the quality of patient care. Funded by the Department of Health, and agreed upon by the UK regulators, it led to a collaborative initiative between the universities of Southampton, Portsmouth and the NHS Strategic Health Authority.

The New Generation Project, initiated by Professor Debra Humphris, now pro vice-chancellor of education at Southampton University, focused on interprofessional learning in undergraduate health and social care programmes across 11 pre-qualifying professions and three foundation degrees (Social Work, Audiology, Nursing, Medicine, Midwifery, Occupational Therapy, Physiotherapy, Podiatry, Pharmacy, Radiography (Diagnostic and Therapeutic)). The main aim of the New Generation Project, one of four leading-edge sites, was to enhance professional competence and so improve the quality of care for patients.

On programme completion, students are expected to demonstrate 'mutual respect for all members of the interprofessional team; a reluctance to stereotype; an absence of discriminatory behaviour; and an increase in their skills and confidence in functioning as an effective interprofessional team member. In addition, graduates should have a better understanding and valuing of the contributions made by others and demonstrate the ability to learn from others in order to benefit service users (patients and clients). Another important aim is to promote an understanding and comfort with different ways of working and changing future professional roles.'[88]

The programme consists of three common learning units, each two weeks in duration and integrated throughout the health and social care curricula (*see* Figure 1.16). While the first unit is campus-based, the two subsequent units involve practice placements with health and social care employers across Hampshire and the Isle of Wight. In the practice placements students are involved in real-world projects (e.g. an audit of hospital admissions procedures), while learning to work effectively together as a team. Annually about 1300 students are divided into small multidisciplinary groups of about 10 students. The three common learning units are as follows.

- Unit 1: Collaborative Learning, based in universities
- Unit 2: Interprofessional Teamworking, based in practice
- Unit 3: Interprofessional Development in Practice, based in practice

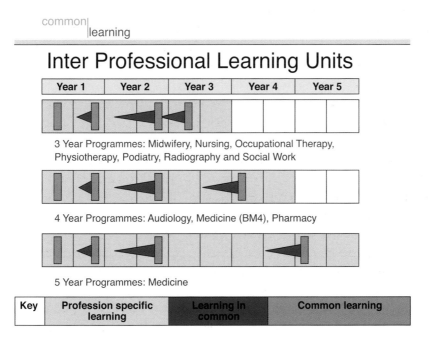

FIGURE 1.16 Interprofessional learning units scheduled across 11 health and social care programmes[88]

The programme has been running since 2001 and continues to make significant progress, to the point that the majority of students indicate they have a positive experience. While generally successful, work remains on identifying group activities that are deemed relevant and 'value-added' by all participating students. In this regard, a future important step would be to broaden the scope of interprofessional and transprofessional education by initiating common learning in both non-clinical *and* clinical areas for health and social care students, as recommended by panel members at the report launch of *Health Professionals for a New Century*.[56] According to the panel members considering transformation of the learning process, 'there are core competencies that all health professions share, which are applicable to all countries despite their resource level' and that '[t]eamwork among the professions can be optimised by shared courses, joint appointments, joint degrees, and interdisciplinary research centers'.[89]

The need for interprofessional education across all disciplines was also emphasised by a University of Michigan taskforce on multidisciplinary learning and team teaching.[90] Possibly speaking for all higher education disciplines that were originally structured to meet the needs of an industrial age, the taskforce declared:

> We believe that the major problems of our time, from the environment to poverty, from human rights to terrorism, from religious movements to healthcare, cannot be studied effectively within any single discipline; all involve integrative thinking. In order to prepare for life of a productive endeavour in the 21st century, graduates … must learn problem-solving across disciplines and launch inquiries in uncharted territories of knowledge and practice. They must examine the assumptions that inhere in a disciplinary perspective and integrate material outside of pattern of thought. … And they must learn how to find their way through disconnected bodies of information and perspectives and create their own path to an education that coheres.

The main issue, as Cathy Davidson,[91] an American university professor and author of *Now You See It: how the brain science of attention will transform the way we live, work, and learn*, asserts in a groundbreaking article is that '[w]e continue to prepare students as if their career path were linear, definite, specialised and predictable. We are making them experts in obsolescence. We are doing a good job of training them for the 20th century.'

However, while interprofessional education or team-based learning appears to be emerging as a priority in several countries, largely because of concerns about patient safety, staff shortages and costs, Dr Lesley Bainbridge, director of Interprofessional Education in the Faculty of Medicine at the University of British Columbia,[92] concludes that progress has been slow despite major changes in healthcare, many of which have been outlined in this chapter. Evidence abounds that we harm patients, and, in social care, clients, when 'we do not

communicate and collaborate both within and among professions'. Bainbridge cites a number of barriers across all professions that undermine integration of interprofessional learning across the professions, including:
- a lack of flexibility in the scheduling of curricular activities
- the challenges of finding space to bring groups of students together
- the costs required for team teaching
- the complexity of assessing students' performance in team teaching settings
- lack of interprofessional placements in the community.

Further, in the practice setting, obstacles to interprofessional learning in healthcare are equally daunting:
- funding to create the organisational changes required to support collaborative or team-based care
- institutional support for a collaborative practice model
- time
- incentives to reinforce best practices in collaboration
- attention to teaching and learning collaborative practice skills as part of continuing professional development.

To this list of obstacles, Gloria Daly, a clinical practice development nurse,[93] adds issues relating to 'the rivalry between professional groups', which Audrey Leathhard[94] describes 'as a form of social Darwinism of occupations'. In addition, another barrier among professional groups might be 'differing moral and ethical philosophies', finances and resource allocation, whereby, for example, 'budget holders are responsible for the education funding of their own professional group', and '[u]nderspend in one's professional group's budget is unlikely to be transferred into another profession's budget irrespective of any educational need to improve patient care'.

The Lancet commissioners would agree with these observations, but add that, while difficult to implement, '[t]eam roles of individual health professionals have floundered amid the divided faculty and curricula of the different professions, the rigid tribalism that afflicts them, hyperspecialisation of some professionals, and overly rigid accreditation standards that restrict opportunities for collaboration'.[56]

Both Bainbridge and Daly seem to concur that an opportunity for significant advancement with interprofessional learning will be provided when 'service delivery is re-designed, especially in areas such as primary health care', which will allow 'a rapidly emerging menu of IPE [interprofessional education] strategies and approaches'. Features these strategies have in common include focusing 'on the learner's attention on patients and families and offer learning experiences in clinically relevant and interesting areas'. Moreover, '[t]hey offer interactive and experiential learning, and they allow time for learners to reflect on their ability to collaborate effectively'. Dr Bainbridge suggests several approaches that institutions may consider in implementing interprofessional learning across healthcare professions:

- student-run clinics
- portfolios
- team-based rural placements
- healthcare team challenges
- joint assessments of patients with complex conditions
- interprofessional problem-based learning sessions.[92]

Moreover, *The Lancet* commissioners assert that 'team learning and interprofessional education cannot be confined to the classroom' and suggest 'greater impact with ancillary modalities including shared seminars in which cross-profession dialogue, joint course work, joint professional volunteering, and interprofessional living-learning accommodation are promoted'. Perhaps, according to the commissioners, even more important for health system performance is transprofessional teamwork that 'includes non-professional health workers ... with basic and ancillary health workers, administrators and managers, policy makers and leaders of the local community'.[56]

Fundamentally, the commissioners assert, 'actual practice in increasingly complex health settings is based on teams' and 'the more the educational experience includes competencies for that type of work, the better health professionals will be equipped to adapt to the teamwork that is imperative of good practice'.[56] As one example of articulating common standards of practice, the Association of Faculties of Medicine of Canada has evolved 'principles and practices for integrating interprofessional education into the accreditation standards for six health professions'.[95] Further, the Canadian Interprofessional Health Collaborative has developed a national competency framework for interprofessional collaboration.[96]

In the United Kingdom the Academy of Medical Royal Colleges and the NHS Institute for Innovation and Improvement, in conjunction with a wide range of stakeholders, have developed the Medical Leadership Competency Framework, which 'describes the leadership competences doctors need in order to become more actively involved in the planning, delivery and transformation of health services'. Built on the concept of shared leadership, the Medical Leadership Competency Framework 'is a pivotal tool which can be used to help design of training curricula and development programmes; highlight individual strengths and development areas through self assessment and structured feedback from colleagues; and help with personal development planning and career progression'.[97]

While there are sceptics – practitioners, students, policymakers – 'there is emerging and robust evidence that interprofessional collaboration does improve patient safety and quality of care as well as improve issues such as recruitment and retention'.[98]

Taking the suggestions of *The Lancet* report, *Health Professionals for a New Century*[56] forward would first require a reconceptualisation of the medical and allied health curricula. Above all, there would need to be much more emphasis on collaborative learning – including clinical skill development – especially in the early years and at core postgraduate levels. In future, it is vital to break down – rather than create – interprofessional barriers, which run counter to 'the notion of interprofessional collective responsibility' and 'professional self-regulation' advocated several years ago by Sir Donald Irvine,[99] then president of the General Medical Council.

Planning and implementing strategies would also necessitate the establishment of government and interprofessional policy groups at national and local levels to tackle the questions that Bainbridge, Daly and others have raised. Fundamental to making the transformation work will be the development of financial models that integrate interprofessional learning in healthcare and that place healthcare providers on a more democratic and equal footing, which may be attractive to government funders, but perhaps less so for some professional bodies.

Moreover, keeping the patient or client as the primary focus of *all* health and social care decisions, and offering more opportunities for learning together interprofessionally, would be consistent with other health and social care directions in several countries, where integration rather than segregation is at the forefront of health and social care planning.

The Lancet commission report and concluding comments

The independent commission of 20 academic leaders from around the world recommended comprehensive reform in the training of healthcare professionals in *Health Professionals for a New Century*.[56]

Paralleling the issues or concerns outlined in this chapter, the report authors confirm that at the beginning of the twenty-first century, there are '[g]laring gaps and inequities in health' that 'persist both within and across countries, underscoring our collective failure to share the dramatic health advances equitably', while new health challenges loom on the horizon. Moreover, the commissioners say, '[p]rofessional education has not kept pace with these challenges, largely because of fragmented, outdated and static curricula that produces ill-equipped graduates. The problems are systemic' and call for '[r]edesign of health education'.

In summary, the main aim of the beginning chapter in this book was to raise awareness of issues – international and national – in the developing and developed world that are impacting on health and medical education in the early years of this century. Subsequent chapters focus on identifying national and international educational priorities and to suggest educational development and change management strategies that may help policymakers, planners and healthcare educationalists to translate proposed reforms and recommendations into reality on the ground. Moreover, later chapters review the role of the medical profession in society and as part of the wider healthcare community. The final chapter draws together and reinforces key considerations and factors in shifting the present 'informative' and 'formative' learning and curriculum models to emerging 'interdependent' healthcare educational paradigms that support the 'transformative' learning of health professionals and the care of patients in the coming decades.[56]

Central to understanding this transformation, and affirmed by *The Lancet* Commission, is the need for a new generation of healthcare professionals, guided by a 'common global vision for the future, where all health professionals in all countries are educated to mobilise knowledge, and to engage in critical reasoning and ethical conduct, so that they are competent to participate in patient-centred and population-centred health systems as members of locally responsive and globally connected teams'. As underscored by the commissioners, '[t]he ultimate purpose of transforming medical education curricula specifically and healthcare curricula generally,' is

> to assure universal coverage of high-quality comprehensive services that are essential to advancing opportunity for health equity within and between countries. The aspiration of good health commonly shared resonates with young professionals who seek value and meaning in their work.[56]

National reviews of medical education

Common issues and concerns in medical education

In the past few years several countries – Australia,[100] Canada[101] and the United States[102–106] – have embarked on reviews of their medical education systems. In the United Kingdom, the General Medical Council has issued its *Education Strategy 2011–2013*,[107] and, more recently, *The State of Medical Education and Practice*,[108] which will become an annual report. While this latter document noted examples of good practice, it also expressed concerns over inconsistencies and variability in healthcare across Britain, insisting that '[m]edical education and training need to be more responsive to changes in healthcare needs, the organisation and delivery of care, and the shifting expectations of patients'. All reports agree that medical education requires vast improvements in order to sustain the changing needs of twenty-first-century society. More specifically, shared curriculum outcomes or common threads include:

- shifting toward competency and outcomes-based education and training models and ensuring greater clarity and consistency of learning outcomes and standards to be met
- individualising the learning experience through more flexible learning (e.g. by allowing 'doctors to move between specialties'[107])
- the view that clinical reasoning ('habits of inquiry'[103]) is best developed by integrating 'fundamental scientific principles, both human and biological sciences in relevant and immediate clinical contexts'
- the recognition that collaborative or inter/trans-professional teamworking[101,102] and a commitment to 'excellence and continuous improvement'[100–106] are at the heart of safe and effective patient care

- that considerable attention needs to be given to working in community settings; formative assessment and feedback;[100] preventive medicine and whole-person integrated curricula, public and global health, professional identity formation and clinical leadership.

National reports and the possible need to 'dig deeper'

While these reports make excellent recommendations for strategic and curriculum change with regard to undergraduate and postgraduate medical education, we may question whether they have gone far enough in addressing more fundamental twenty-first-century health and social care issues and setting out more detailed 'enabling actions' backed by objective data.

- Is healthcare safe? Equitable?[56]
- If not, what needs to be done differently?
- What changes to governance and professional development are necessary?
- What are the long-term social and health implications of an ageing society?
- How are governments tackling obesity, diabetes, musculoskeletal disorders, respiratory diseases, cardiovascular diseases, cancer, chronic kidney disease and other illnesses?[49]
- How does effectiveness of treatments compare across the country and the world?
- What are the causes of variance and how do costs compare?
- What structural and process changes are required to shift from the biomedical model of illness, which has dominated healthcare for over a century, to a preventive model of care?
- To what extent have previous studies into healthcare effectiveness and efficiency made a difference to the quality of patient care?
- Can we learn from other paradigmatic societal changes where successful paradigm shifts have occurred (e.g. technology and the internet)?
- What can be done to encourage more people to take personal responsibility for their health and well-being?
- How do we support patients to make positive behavioural changes?
- How can enabling actions be supported so that transformations actually do take place?
- In other words, what have we learned about the management of change in the last few decades that may help steer a path through the network of complex healthcare structures and policies, organisations and vested interests?

Surely, one lesson is that good intentions and eloquent rhetoric – as we have seen pursuant to many natural disasters and healthcare interventions[7] – do not provide a guarantee that things will change and that it takes a certain kind of leadership to help transition from political goodwill to helpful developmental initiatives that actually make a difference in people's lives. In addition, while all reports have considered recommendations, what some reports fail to discuss in greater depth is the moral responsibility of high-income nations to the developing world, with over five billion people, and the details of the healthcare support that is urgently needed, as is clear from patient-to-doctor ratios.[77] The importance of this interdependency was most recently highlighted in the 2010 international *The Lancet*-commissioned report *Health Professionals for a New Century: transforming education to strengthen health systems in an interdependent world*,[56] chaired by Professor Julio Frenk, dean of Harvard's School of Public Health and co-chaired by Dr Lincoln Chen, president of the China Medical Board.

Balancing primary care and the specialties

Over the past four decades, expansion in hospital services, triggered largely by 'rapid scientific and technological advance' and the growth of sub-specialisations, has also become a cause for concern. As Sir Donald Irvine, then president of the General Medical Council, asked several years ago, in the future will it be possible 'to hold medicine together as a distinctive entity?'[99]

Given today's financial strains, it appears likely that radical change is required in order to sustain the beneficial role that the specialties within medicine provide. Professor Paul Corrigan, former policy advisor for the Department of Health, says that hospitals will close in the UK as the NHS desperately seeks to make savings.[109] His main argument is that each year demand for NHS services increases largely because of an ageing population, with the increase in demand estimated at about 20% in the next five years while public financing will rise by just 1%. Further, he advises, '[a]s with every other industry or service, the NHS will have to provide improvements with the same resources'. This challenge can only be achieved by '[s]pecialisation and the division of labour' in order to 'improve the efficiency of all services and industries'. In other words, '[i]f you have one hospital performing 1,000 procedures, it is much more efficient than ten hospitals each carrying out 100. If every local hospital tries to do everything, we need to have much bigger subsidies to keep them going so inefficiently.' According to Professor Corrigan, the choice for the UK government – and possibly other governments also – is '[e]ither support local hospitals to reduce radically the range of services they offer or find a lot of extra money for their inefficiency – and still watch some hospitals fail completely'.

If district hospitals focus on specialised services, there may be implications for both specialist and GP care. One implication is that the hospitals would no longer be able to provide the whole range of specialty services but would instead have to focus on high-risk conditions or common surgical procedures, such as cardiac care or hernias. Another is that changes along these lines will likely lead to greater choice for patients, competition for treatment, which could drive up quality care, and transparency of information. Professor Sir Bruce Keogh, NHS medical director and past president of the Society for Cardiothoracic Surgery,[110] gives the example of stroke services in London, saying that at one point [before February 2010] 32 hospitals provided immediate stroke treatment. However, it is recognised that 'stroke treatment is complex and potentially risky', and that not all hospitals could provide adequate services to treat emergency situations [over 11 000 people in London suffer a stroke every year]. To improve stroke services, it was agreed that the number of emergency treatment facilities should be reduced to eight and that they be located in areas where ambulances could easily reach them. Results to date 'show that four times as many patients are treated with clot-busting drugs, reducing disability; that there is less variation in death rates around the capital and patients spend less time in hospital'. Also, some of the procedures currently provided in hospitals may be made available locally through polyclinics, mini-invasive treatment centres (e.g. laparascopic and endovascular procedures) or general practice surgeries, with much enhanced technological diagnostic and treatment support.

In the UK, and perhaps other countries, future specialisation may focus more on extending the skill set of GPs – possibly following the US model of training 'internal medicine specialists or internists who specialise in primary and comprehensive care of adults and adolescents and are at the forefront of managing chronic diseases'.[111] Rebalancing is required not only between hospital and community-based practice but also between specialisations and general practice, which, as in the United States, may need to undergo major review and readjustment or restructuring to remain viable. As the demand for services – especially with regard to chronic diseases and social care – increases, there is the real possibility that some services may go bankrupt. In some countries, there is a case to be made for greater efficiency and effectiveness by creating, as two examples, new professional roles, such as 'assistant physicians,' an intermediate position between nurses and physicians, or 'community health and social care support workers,' with hybrid responsibilities that holistically maximise individual patient care.

In an interesting report on the state of the NHS, part of a wider investigation of how to 'fix' the NHS, Camilla Cavendish, lead writer for *The Times*,[112] and journalist Alex Ralph interviewed about 100 health practitioners across the UK about how well the system was working. An excerpt from this report is cause for concern and highlights that there are significant variations in the quality of care across the country and that considerable improvements are a matter of urgency.

Care in Britain ranges from world-class to shocking. Between 1998 and 2006, 1.6% of bowel cancer sufferers died within a month at the Manchester Royal Infirmary, compared with 15.6% at Queen's Hospital, Burton upon Trent. The National Lung Cancer audit has just reported a sixfold difference in the proportion of lung cancer patients receiving potentially life-saving surgery in different parts of the country in 2009: 31% at Barts, London, and only 5% of patients at the Shrewsbury and Telford Hospital NHS Trust. And Lord Darzi of Denham famously reported that Westminster and Canning Town were separated by eight stops on the Jubilee Line, but by a seven-year disparity in life expectancy. That is unacceptable.

At a recent dinner, one clinical director told colleagues that he had chosen to undergo an operation at his own hospital. The majority of the other clinical directors said that they wouldn't dream of choosing their own hospital. If they don't trust it, they shouldn't ask the rest of us to.

While also finding some situations of 'madness', they also identified many examples of excellence and innovative practice that provided improvements without requiring a change in the law. Cavendish cites the Royal Free Hospital in London, where Dr John Horton, 'an enterprising local GP, explains that he has persuaded the hospital to create a sort of front parlour, where two GPs see 1,000 people a week and treat about 450. They do suturing, X-rays, and blood tests without using up precious time of hospital doctors.' Cavendish refers to another case where the GPs assessed an elderly patient with pneumonia, fixed him up with intravenous antibiotics and sent a nurse home with him. The tension between hospital and community care was well summarised in Cavendish's report by a quote from Dr Howard Stoate, a GP and an ex-member of parliament: 'To us GPs it makes sense to do our own cardiac scans in our surgery. To a hospital finance director, it doesn't.'

Cavendish also asked the question, 'How good are our GPs?' and concluded that '[a]ccording to the OECD, they are now the highest paid in the world', largely because of the 2004 contract, which 'effectively paid them more to do less, giving bonuses for flu shots, and ditching out-of-hours cover with over [f]orty percent of GPs (who) are now salaried [many part-time women], not independent contractors ... with the average GP spending only 22.5 hours a week with patients. That might explain why they are always rushed and can see you only for eight minutes.' One reason for the increasing costs of hospital care was offered by another London GP: 'If the patients can't get a GP, they go to Accident and Emergency [A&E]. Receptionists routinely advise people to go to a walk-in centre at 4:00 p.m. in the afternoon.' Her own recommendations for improving healthcare – the Cavendish Recommendations – some of which may resonate with other health systems, include drawing 'up a new GP contract with round-the-clock responsibility'; elevating 'basic care skills in nursing'; regulating 'healthcare assistants'; letting 'other providers take over failing hospitals'; encouraging 'specialisation'; encouraging 'competition in community services'; printing 'prices on drugs/equipment to show they are not free'; trusting 'patients with their medical records, and digitise them'; making 'GP commissioning optional, not compulsory; and creating proper lines of authority'.

Cavendish and Ralph also tried to determine the root causes undermining the UK NHS: Money? Structure? Management? Some of these may have parallels in other health systems. One of their key findings[112] was that '[c]ontrary to popular myth, the NHS is not a "monolith",' but rather 'about 700 fatally disconnected organisations, Hospitals, GPs, and community health services with separate budgets, management structures and information systems. Our test results, our appointments, our care can fall into the cracks.'

Further, they observe, '[t]he system is full of perverse incentives with Britain sending more people to hospital per head of population than any other country, except Austria, partly because the Government pays hospitals by activity, not outcome'. They then conclude – along with the present UK government – that the current situation cannot continue, 'because of a fundamental change which is taking place in our society. Diseases that might have carried someone off ten years ago – diabetes, heart disease, dementia – are now "long-term conditions" that need treating outside of hospital.'

In Sweden, Bertil Hamberger,[113] professor emeritus of molecular medicine and surgery at Karolinska Institutet, observed several years ago that '[r]eorganisations and closings of smaller hospitals are continually occurring, and various organisational models are being tested.' Further, he noted that small hospitals in urban areas needed 'to undergo structural changes, subspecialisation, mergers, or closure'. These changes would also have a knock-on effect on the future training of doctors, as GPs may have to boost their skill levels and surgeons may require broader training to work in smaller centres. While speculative, there may be a decrease or mergers in specialties, although the influx of migrants and increasingly older patients may lessen this possibility.

The story is similar in the United States with regard to general practice, where, for instance, '[t]here are approximately 269,000 primary care physicians. ... Of those, about 38 percent are family physicians' compared with approximately 50% in 1961.[114] In terms of medical education, and in line with World Health Organization[11] recommendations, the American Academy of Family Physicians (AAFP), while trying to avoid a crisis, recommends that '[m]edical school expansion must be developed in ways that target primary care rural and underserved practice'. The AAFP also argues for providing '[f]inancial incentives to medical schools that consistently produce higher numbers of primary care physicians'. One of the reasons that US physicians choose the path of specialisation is simply the cost of medical education and the ability to repay loans – which will now also become a serious issue in the UK, with tuition fees for most undergraduate education rising to over £9000 starting in 2012.

Prompted by a concern about the shortage of primary care physicians, with estimates ranging from 44 000 to 46 000 by 2025, major changes are also taking place in the United States. Here a key report, entitled *Ensuring an Effective Physician Workforce for America: recommendations for an accountable graduate medical education system*,[103] released in February 2011, 'urged Congress to seek an independent, external review of how U.S. graduate medical education programs are governed, financed, and regulated'. The overall aim of the report, led by '[a] panel of leaders in academic medicine and health care' and whose recommendations received nearly $10 billion in federal support, is to ensure America is 'producing the right number and mix of physicians and that they are more accountable to public need'.[103]

The report's major recommendations included calling for a review of the governance and financing of the current graduate medical education (GME) system and paying special attention 'to clinical experience requirements and length of training'. The report also questioned the need 'of the transitional year program or preliminary year experiences required by some specialties' and emphasised the importance of beginning 'a process that encourages and promotes innovative training approaches and creation of new GME programs to better serve the needs of the public and better prepare trainees for a rapidly changing practice environment'.

In a quick response, the 2010 report was closely followed in late 2011 by *Ensuring an Effective Physician Workforce for the United States: recommendations for reforming graduate medical education to meet the needs of the public*,[104] which recommends major changes in the way residents are trained to meet public needs. These recommendations include:

- *Making 'graduate medical education more accountable to the public'*. As GME 'is financed with public dollars' there is a need 'to create and maintain an ongoing exchange with the public', including 'the voice of the public' on 'boards and committees of institutions that sponsor GME and the organizations that oversee it'.
- *Replacing 'time-based training with outcomes-based standards that link graduation to readiness for unsupervised practice'*. Further, '[t]he group says that the current system of training all residents for a fixed duration "fails to recognise or accommodate" the reality that residents vary in how quickly they achieve competency'. Moreover, '[t]he panel recommends moving from measuring months and years of training to a system based on an individual's readiness for independent practice', and by '[r]outinely aligning the duration of training to individual residents' achievement of competence would yield a more consistent level of skills among physicians entering unsupervised practice,

more efficient delivery of competent practitioners to the public, and more responsible use of public funding supporting resident education'.

- *Expanding 'the content and sites of training to reflect current and future patient needs … with an urgency to more effectively deliver an updated curriculum, in part by diversifying the training sites for GME* (including federally quali-fied health centres and school-based health centres, for example) to provide a breadth of clinical experience beyond traditional teaching hospitals and to expand content related to professionalism, population medicine, and team-based practice'. In terms of competencies, '[t]he group says ACGME's [Accreditation Council for Graduate Medical Education] core competencies must be better integrated with clinical performance since they "remain poorly standardized and incompletely assessed and are too often taught and evaluated outside the context of patient care"'.

- *Encouraging 'collaborative education', advocating 'for the elimination of histori-cal professional boundaries so that inter-specialty and inter-professional education become a consistent element of physician training'*. In addition, it is felt that 'all residents should have the opportunity to learn with and from physician colleagues in other specialties and other health professionals', necessitat-ing 'revising regulations that now prevent supervision across specialties or professions'.[111]

Targeting 'medical educators and leaders of institutions that train residents, and at groups that set the standards such as the Accreditation Council for Graduate Medical Education and American Board of Medical Specialties', the report authors recommend the 'creation of a National Institute of Health Professions Education to fund and coordinate research efforts across multiple sites and health professions'. Establishing this Institute, it is believed, 'will result in more productive and cost-effective research, urgently needed to guide improvements in physician and health professions training'.[104]

These major new directions will greatly influence, as detailed in later chap-ters of this book, how we need to reconceptualise and deliver the training of all healthcare professionals. For example, in the UK, because more will need to be done locally, requiring additional skills and technological support, core training may become lengthier[107] and much more interprofessionally and transprofession-ally team-oriented,[56,101,104] with some specialisation possibly occurring at specific organ or disease levels.

Largely because of cost containment, training timelines may need to be made more flexible, using outcomes-based rather than cohort time-limited or standard rotations[104] or clinical placements, or even reduced with more opportunities provided for students and junior doctors for early patient contact and practising some medicine under close supervision. In the future, consideration may be given to modularised healthcare training, whereby healthcare students could proceed through the same modules with certificated stepping-off points, allowing the trainees to practise in a professional capacity and with new emerging job descriptions (e.g. cardio support practitioner) in a defined area under supervision with the possibility of returning to take further modules and advancing toward more complex training and posts. These directions are in keeping with the increasing blurring of roles and overlapping responsibilities.

These changes, if predictions are accurate, may not sit well with some conservative elements of society, but they may provide a necessary bridge – where medicine has become largely unaffordable, dehumanised, with a demoralised workforce and variable outcomes – to one that is more affordable, personalised with happier employees and more consistent results across community-driven healthcare.

Barriers to achieving reforms

Responding to *The Lancet* report, Patrick Lee *et al.*[115] identified two main barriers in the United States – and most likely these are barriers in other countries too – to achieving reforms. One is the 'underemphasis of health systems in the standard curriculum', while the other relates to the 'artificial separation of global health and primary care'. As one response, the Massachusetts General Hospital, a major teaching hospital of Harvard Medical School, developed a new internal medicine residency programme in global primary care 'to bridge global health and primary care', integrating 'the standard clinical curriculum with a public health degree and longitudinal primary care systems training in both urban USA and rural Uganda'.[115]

Other hurdles to implementing the reforms, outlined by a panel at *The Lancet* report launch, 'include the conservative nature of universities and their department-based structures, credentialing and reward systems; most university leaders don't feel an incentive to change; and there is currently no model to aspire to'.[116] Most panel members also agreed that 'it will take strong leadership to transform the learning environment at the regulatory and accreditation level, within professional societies, and among health professional faculties', and while '[p]roblems with health education worldwide are similar … solutions will have to be national or regional, although lessons can be learned from each other's efforts'.

Educational priorities in medical education

A synthesis of key educational priorities in medical education

Figure 3.1 summarises priorities for medical education in the next decade drawn from multiple sources, including national reports – Australia,[100] Canada,[101] the US,[102–106] and the United Kingdom[107,108] – as well as drawing on other papers,[117,118] categorised under three main headings: systemic factors, curriculum and learning.

Systemic problems in medical education

Systemic issues call for better balance and integration of a number of curriculum aspects with greater emphasis on preventive medicine, collaboration, and public and global health with improvements to educational resources including consideration for localising medical and social care. In terms of training physicians, they also have a management planning and human resource dimension. As decision-making will increasingly move toward local communities, physicians and other professionals will need to become more knowledgeable about resource planning, working with structures and organisations that may also support localised patient and social care. Educational research to evaluate progress and identify potential solutions should become a built-in requirement of all initiatives.[104] Echoing findings from the World Health Organization 2008 World Health Report,[56] the 20 professional and academic leaders of *The Lancet*-commissioned report *Health Professionals for a New Century: transforming education to strengthen health systems in an interdependent world*[56] conclude that the problems with twenty-first-century healthcare education are also mostly systemic (*see* Figure 3.2).

Systemic	Curriculum	Learning
• Shifting from hospital to community-based training and expanding clinical sites • Placing more emphasis on population needs • Putting the patient at the centre • Implementing information systems (local/global) • Balancing curative and preventive medicine • Understanding cultural differences – traditions, treatments and so forth • Enhancing collaborative learning and teamworking • Putting more emphasis on public and global health • Improving quality and access to resources • Localising health and social care responsibilities • Supporting patient opportunities for choice in treatment • Encouraging physicians to learn about resource planning and working effectively in complex structures and systems • Nurturing an effective and sustainable workforce and rebalancing the labour market • Ensuring gender equity • Developing healthcare leadership • Ensuring transparency and openness	• Ensuring the curriculum is socially accountable • Ensuring the curriculum is competency and outcomes based (versus time based) • Integrating technical and complex adaptive competencies • Ensuring competencies meet the needs of the patients and that learning outcomes are clear and user-friendly • Improving the integration of science and clinical, science and humanities • Addressing the hidden curriculum • Ensuring assessments match competencies and learning outcomes and provide opportunities for self and peer assessments • Ensuring that feedback is timely and helpful	• Implementing active learning based on constructivist learning principles (i.e. personal 'meaning making') • Fostering clinical reasoning and 'habits of inquiry' • Recognising the importance of both the art and science of healthcare • Questioning senior staff and consultants without fear of intimidation • Providing opportunities for individualised and small group learning • Encouraging use of multi-mediated learning • Participating in leadership development

Engaging in Healthcare Education Research and Evidence-Based Practice

FIGURE 3.1 A synthesis of educational priorities in healthcare education

According to the international authors of the report, 'changes are needed because of fragmented, outdated, and static curricula that produce ill-equipped doctors, nurses, midwives, and public health professionals'.[119] As summarised in Figure 3.3, the Commission

> calls for a broad reform movement, encompassing instructional design (what we teach and how) and institutional design (schools or universities that should

Systemic failures
- Mismatch of competencies to needs
- Weak teamwork
- Gender stratification
- Hospital dominance over primary care
- Labour market imbalances
- Weak leadership for health system performance

FIGURE 3.2 *The Lancet* report: system failures

carry out instruction). In terms of instructional design, the approach should be competency-based and inter-professional, bringing together health professionals to work as a cohesive team. It should use information technology (IT) to empower health professionals during training and in the field.[56]

On the other hand, to improve healthcare education through institutional design,

much tighter coordination is needed between education and the health sector to ensure that the type of health professionals trained matches the health needs in every country. In addition, global coalitions, associations and networks are needed to better leverage educational resources from around the world. With the aim of developing transformative and interdependent professional education, the authors have also identified four key enabling actions or strategies.[56]

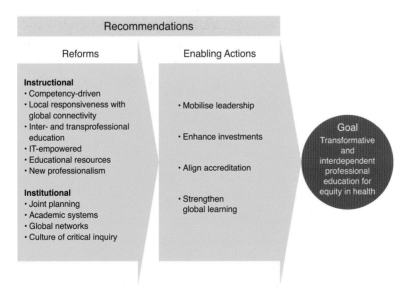

FIGURE 3.3 *The Lancet* report: summary of reforms and enabling actions[56]

Curriculum reform in medical education: returning to first principles?

While acknowledging major challenges, the authors of *The Lancet*-commissioned report are arguing for a radical restructuring of healthcare education curricula. To minimise fragmentation, ensure greater relevance and give the study of medicine the momentum for change it requires, healthcare bodies and educators across the globe might be prudent to start their reconceptualisation almost from a *tabula rasa* perspective. The suggested 'Competency, Integration, Inter/transprofessionalism and Creativity' (*CIIC*) framework (*see* Chapter 4 for outline) could be helpful in considering fundamental design components. In a sense, the changes being called for – although much wider in scope and magnitude and potentially involving all healthcare professions – are as fundamental or groundbreaking as those introduced by Sir William Osler (1849–1919)[120] and Abraham Flexner (1866–1959)[121] in medical education in the early years of the twentieth century. These two contemporaries probably did for medical education what Louis Pasteur (1822–95)[122] and Robert Koch (1843–1910)[123] did for medical science in the late nineteenth century.

After making major contributions to medical education at McGill University in Canada and Johns Hopkins University in the United States, Sir William Osler, a Canadian physician, author and educator, assumed the post of Regius Professor of Medicine at Oxford University in 1905, 'at the time the most prestigious medical appointment in the English-speaking world'.[120] Placing the microscope at the centre of medical education and with his emphasis on small group teaching, clinical clerkships and patient contact, he changed medical education in the late nineteenth and early twentieth centuries. Among his many accomplishments is the publication in 1892 of what many consider to be 'the most important English medical textbook for a generation of doctors, *The Principles and Practice of Medicine*'.[124] The book, which 'supported his imaginative new curriculum … was based upon the advances in medical science of the previous fifty years'.[120] In addition, 'Osler introduced the German postgraduate training system, instituting one year of general internship followed by several years of residency with increasing clinical responsibilities'.[120] Considered collectively, Osler 'revolutionised the medical curriculum of the United States and Canada, synthesizing the best of the English and German systems'.[120]

Similarly, the US educator Abraham Flexner's report on *Medical Education in the United States and Canada* (1910)[125] 'was monumental in helping to define excellence for the next century of medical education'.[126] Sharing many of Osler's concerns, Flexner 'taught that students learn best through activity of mind and body rather than the traditional "bookish" learning and daily recitation'. Thomas Neville Bonner observes that 'America owes to Flexner, more than any other person, the rapid implementation of the full-time medical school, allied to a teaching hospital and integrated into a university'.[121] Further, Bonner notes, '[i]t was he who defined what a medical school should and should not be'. His emphasis on 2 years' preclinical scientific studies, followed by 2 years of formal clinical education and clerkships or firms, became the universal pattern of medical education throughout the world. His reforms were subsequently agreed and implemented by medical bodies in the United States, Canada and Britain. Further, he 'extended his study of medical education to the German Empire, Austria, and France'. However, his influence went beyond western Europe, as the Flexner model was translated into action through the establishment of new medical schools, the earliest and most prominent being the Peking Union Medical College founded in China by the Rockefeller Foundation and implemented by its China Medical Board in 1917.[56]

Bonner recognises that Flexner 'was one of a small number of persons, such as the British John Maynard Keynes in economic matters and William Beveridge in unemployment and health policy, and the American Wilbur Cohen in health and social legislation, who moved across intellectual boundaries while working with great organisations'. These well-known individuals 'stimulated new approaches to the great policy questions facing health, science, education and welfare in the modern age'. Also '[i]t was Flexner's genius to create and implement new models of organisation to improve education, train better doctors, and bring science into the hospitals.' Bonner notes that '[i]n this respect he was a very modern figure who combined real intellectual power with vision and action in the public sphere'.[121] In many respects, we are at the same place as Flexner was more than 100 years ago, but the world has changed dramatically since then and, given the plight of the developing world and the present assumptions of the developed, we must change with it.

Main purpose of restructuring healthcare education and training

There can be no doubt that many of the issues and questions that Osler and Flexner tackled over a hundred years ago remain with us today. Consider the following examples:
- How are scientific principles best joined to clinical problem-solving and liberal knowledge?
- What part in training should be spent in learning about disease prevention and health promotion, what part about treating illness?
- How is new scientific knowledge best incorporated in the curriculum?
- Can politics and vested interests be kept out of curriculum requirements?[117]

Given these and other policy and curriculum-related questions, one of the central aims of the present recommendations for restructuring[56] – and, indeed, a major purpose of this book – would be to find the best ways of organising not just the medical but all healthcare curricula to ensure that the needs of patients in the twenty-first century are met in the most caring and financially affordable manner. Many of the pieces – medical and pedagogical – of the jigsaw already exist but require rethinking, reprioritising and reshaping by committed stakeholders, with a view to developing more alternatives in terms of structures, flexibility in learning and learner support.

In terms of content, greater priority would likely need to be given to balancing technical and adaptive skills (with emphasis on caring for the elderly), curative and preventive health, hospital and community care, uniprofessionalism and interprofessionalism, science and the humanities, along with considering global and multicultural aspects.

At postgraduate medical training levels, trainees will in the future probably need to devote more of their time between community (e.g. polyclinics, care homes) urban and rural and hospital care, and it will be important 'to pro vide challenge and to build skills and gain experience without hazarding patient safety'. To minimise confusion resulting from multisite working and to ensure trainees benefit from robust and balanced clinical experiences, consideration may need to be given to more managed or deliberate, perhaps longitudinal, rotations – especially at core levels.[102] For example, the authors of a recent study on the current rotational model suggest that '[c]linical experiences should be designed to facilitate learning in a manner that allows the trainee to function as part of an effective interprofessional team that works together longitudinally to resolve meaningful problems'.[128] More recently, there is also considerable attention being given to outcomes-based learning and individualising the trainee learning experience as trainees enter clinical environments with different levels of skills, interests or experience.[104]

Competencies for the twenty-first century

Teamwork is vital, as Richard Smith, a physician, and former editor of the *BMJ*, observes. Physicians are frequently confronted with 'unclear patient problems with unclear solutions', and trying to use technical skills, when answers may lie with applying non-technical or adaptive skills.[129] His basic argument is that, along with technical skills, medical education should incorporate understanding and applying the 'tools and mindset needed to facilitate processes in human systems'. The importance of recognising basic human factors – in particular, face-to-face communication, a key adaptive skill – in supporting patients is highlighted by

Phil Hammond, a UK physician, journalist, comic and broadcaster. He makes the point that 'since the Black report in 1980, we have known that the causes of ill-health are social and so are the solutions'. While tongue in cheek, yet also serious, he concludes that '[i]f you have no job, no home, and no future, you up the heroin and skimp on the oily fish'. His key message is that 'we need self-esteem and an optimistic future before we'll take responsibility for our health and stop overloading the NHS'.[130] In the immediate future his message will be difficult to fulfil. Along similar lines, according to Liz Miller, matron at Queen Elizabeth Hospital in Birmingham, UK, 'a [t]rick they [the Government] are missing is the integration of health and social care budgets. We can get someone fit, but if they live on their own they need help. We have no access to that budget.'[112]

Difficulties experienced by some physicians working in current environments might also be traced back to their previous education and training. As Cathy Davidson[91] observes, '[o]ur educational systems, so far, look as if the internet hasn't been invented yet'. She further concludes that '[t]he history of 20th-century higher education has been the history of assessing individual achievement, measuring, certifying and quantifying outcomes and outputs'. She asks us to '[t]hink about the skills' the twenty-first century 'environment requires', including 'new sorting and attentional skills, collaborative skills, judgement and logical skills, synthesising and analytical abilities, critical and creative skills, qualitative and quantitative skills, all together, with few lines between them. These are sometimes called "21st-century literacies", a range of new interpersonal, synthesising, organising and communication skills that companies insist today's graduates lack.' These integrative competencies or 'intellectual complex adaptive skills', as David Bennet,[131] an expert in knowledge management and organisational development, calls them, 'provide the connective tissue, creating the knowledge, skills, abilities and behaviors that support and enhance other competencies [and] have a multiplier effect through their capacity to enrich the individual's cognitive abilities while enabling integration of other competencies, leading to improved understanding, performance and decisions'.

Refocusing medical education: from teaching to learning

From a historical perspective, the authors of *Health Professionals for a New Century: transforming education to strengthen health systems in an interdependent world*[56] identify three major 'generations of educational reforms' (*see* Figure 3.4) during the twentieth century: a science-based curriculum at the turn of the century, problem-based learning approaches in the latter half of the twentieth century and now recommend a systems-based third generation approach 'to improve the

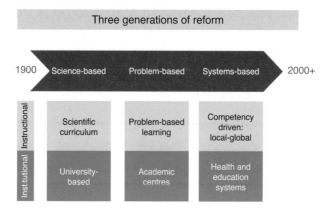

FIGURE 3.4 *The Lancet* report: three generations of reforms[56]

performance of health systems by adapting core professional competencies to specific contexts, while drawing on global knowledge'.

The longer-term view is to 'assure universal coverage of the high-quality comprehensive services that are essential to advance opportunity for health equity within and between countries'. To accomplish these goals the authors propose two fundamental outcomes: (1) transformative learning and (2) interdependence in education. Moving from 'informative (skills) to formative (values) to transformative learning (leadership)' would require

> shifts from fact memorisation to searching, analysis, and synthesis of information for decision making; from seeking professional credentials to achieving core competencies for effective teamwork in health systems; and from non-critical adoption of educational models to creative adaptation of global resources to address local priorities.

The authors' vision of learning – which builds on constructivist influences, whereby 'the world that the learner knows is a world which the learner constructs',[132,133] could facilitate a more harmonious integration of knowledge and understanding of science and the humanities, professional attitudes, and clinical experience – all of which have been major points of contention in medical education at least since the early nineteenth century.

Considering Confucian and Socratic learning philosophies

In developing nations, the challenge may be quite different. In this regard differing societal values and educational systems will mean situating proposed reforms in local contexts.[56] This respect for differences can also be generalised for approaches to study. As Tweed and Lehman[134] note, 'Socrates valued private and public questioning of widely accepted knowledge and expected students to generate and consider their own hypothesis'. On the other hand, Confucius 'valued effortful, respectful, absorptive and pragmatic learning and poetic ambiguity'. The authors' observation that '[i]deally, in our increasingly multicultural world students would be able to competently exhibit a range of both Confucian and Socratic learning behaviours' seems timely and appropriate. In the longer term, both Western and Eastern cultures may come to realise that they have much to gain from each other in terms of educational philosophies, and, broadly speaking, understanding the difference between valuing 'the inner' and 'the outer' life'.[135]

Educational challenges in implementing 'transformative' learning

While there are likely many political challenges in implementing healthcare reforms, from a practical standpoint, at least in the developed world, there may also be fundamental educational challenges that require resolution if 'transformative learning' is to become more pervasive. The central issue relates to the long-standing university tradition – reinforced in the nineteenth century by the German universities and in the twentieth century by scientific research, which prizes the 'logical scientific' paradigm above all others. This insistence may be responsible, arguably, for delays in making human progress, which essentially involves 'making something new'; learning 'how to make the same thing more cheaply'; or 'learning how to make the same thing better'.[2]

Achieving these ends generally requires making sense of the world on a personal level or personal 'meaning-making' (constructivism) that is optimised through reflective practice,[136] and not necessarily based on implicit beliefs that all problems have a scientific solution. Peter Senge at the Massachusetts Institute of Technology, and founding chair of the Society for Organizational Learning, succinctly expresses the damaging impact of the latter Positivist epistemology on students:

> Individualism and competition still reign, from individual students pitted against one another to individual professors who likewise compete for status, power and often money. 'Technical rationality' still ranks as the prevailing epistemology, disconnecting theory from practice and sending young people into the world with heads full of ideas and 'answers' but little experience in producing more effective action.[137]

Dictating what is researched, the questions and interpretation of results, the scientific paradigm, according to the philosopher, Thomas Kuhn, 'does not progress towards truths, but is subject to dogma and clinging to old theories'.[138] The paradigm, closely related to the Aristotelian view of knowledge – what something is rather than what it might become, the Platonic belief, also seems to influence expectations about the educational experience of incoming medical students, many of whom, for example, feel more comfortable with clinically related topics (the science of medicine) rather than the human side of healing, possibly forgetting one of the wise teachings attributed to Hippocrates: 'It's far more important to know what person the disease has than what disease the person has.' In addition, it seems that too much learning is still based on note-taking, memorising facts and not analysis, questioning or probing beyond what is 'in the book' and responding to examination questions that demand formulaic responses rather than empathetic and creative thought and that consider the patient as an individual, who has not only physical but also emotional needs. However, these behaviours may be out of step, as Senge[137] posits, with the students actually being able to apply that learning in a timely and useful fashion, including transference of knowledge into clinical contexts.

The recent UK General Medical Council report *The State of Medical Education and Practice*[108] 'describes the current composition of the medical profession, and demographic trends over time', including some interesting findings on gender, ethnicity and age, including:

- increasing number and proportion of female doctors
- most commonly, doctors are in their early 30s
- more than a third of registered doctors completed their primary medical qualification outside the UK
- the medical profession is more ethnically diverse compared with the UK's general population
- medical specialties, in which doctors work, vary enormously in size and are not always aligned to service needs.

While these findings are important, as they identify trends and draw our attention to potential concerns, more information about the profile of medical practitioners would also be helpful. Knowing more about incoming students' personality traits can help us to better understand their preferences in terms of learning, career specialisation, patient interaction and preferences for clinical environments. More specifically, several studies have used the Myers-Briggs personality profile inventory to help in student selection as the inventory, which has high face validity,[139] can be useful in finding out 'how medical students are energised, how they take data in and process it, how they make decisions, and how they prefer to live their lives on a day-to-day basis'. The inventory can show student preference[140,141] for **E**xtraversion (versus **I**ntroversion), **T**hinking (versus **I**ntuition), **S**ensing (versus **F**eeling) and **J**udging (versus **P**erceiving). Their preference for use of the senses, logic and finishing tasks may make adopting more flexible approaches to change and innovation in medical practice difficult for some. What is also noteworthy and slightly worrying is that

> [c]ompared with data from the 1950s, the type distribution of physicians has remained fairly stable, save for *a trend toward more judging types*. Women in medicine today are more representative of the general population on the feeling dimension than earlier, when medicine was more male-dominated. Women are more likely than men to choose primary care specialties, as are those with preference for introversion and feeling. Feeling types choose Family Medicine significantly more often than thinking types; male, extraverted, and thinking types choose surgical specialties. Of those selecting nonprimary care, male, extraverted, and thinking types choose surgical specialties significantly more than women, introverted, and feeling types.[140]

At trainee or resident levels, a study at Temple University also found similar correlations between personality preferences and choice of medical specialty.[142] Many of the specialties were dominated by Judgers, including paediatrics, anaesthesiology and orthopaedics. Interestingly, psychiatry was the only specialty where Perceivers were the majority. Perceivers, who are direct opposites of Judgers – are supposed to be spontaneous, easy-going, adaptable and more open to change – arguably key characteristics expected of healthcare professionals in the twenty-first century. While requiring further research, the data to date may have implications for student selection, where more weight might be given to those who demonstrate empathy, adaptability and openness to change.

Greater emphasis on working in interprofessional healthcare teams and interactions in multidisciplinary social settings are certainly two ways forward in preparing future health and social care professionals.

Enhancing understanding and acquisition of professional skills

In tune with Donald Schön's work,[136] some may agree that there are limitations on applying principles of technical rationality, which assumes that theoretical knowledge must be the foundation of practice, to education and the professional development of health professionals. Indeed there may be a case to be made that the technical-rational 'discourse', based largely on research-generated and systemised knowledge, actually inhibits the development of 'habits of inquiry'.[102]

Dall'Alba and Sandberg[143] note that 'most contemporary models of skill development were devised within cognitive psychology', generally identifying attributes in a decontextualized manner – 'an approach that reflects a container view of practice' – with skill acquisition occurring in stages from novice to expert levels. In their review the authors critique stage models as they could veil 'more fundamental aspects of development' by directing attention away from the skill being developed and that 'a fundamental dimension of professional skill building is overlooked' – namely, 'understanding of, and in, practice', developed over time.

Their alternative model proposes a horizontal and vertical dimension to professional development. The horizontal dimension would encompass traditional skill development, whereas the vertical dimension would call 'attention to variation in embodied understanding of practice'. In medicine, for example, doctors 'may devote most of their working lives to refining an existing understanding' but not necessarily 'transformation in embodied understanding of medical practice (along the vertical axis)', such as deciding to provide a better balance to illness prevention and cure.

In terms of education, the authors advocate creating 'opportunities for learning that both call into question and extend participants' current understanding of, and in, practice'. Dall'Aba and Sandberg's research highlights the importance of careful monitoring of trainee performance and focusing – in keeping with transformative learning principles – on their 'understanding', of the practice, not just the technical or procedural skills involved, and to discuss implications for their training or the programme generally. Citing other studies, the authors conclude that 'professional development involves not simply accumulating knowledge and skills, but learning to deal with the situations encountered in qualitatively different and complex ways'. They caution that '[e]fforts of this kind are likely to be successful only when the focus throughout a course or program is on the development of such understanding'.

Two conclusions seem to stand out from this notable study: first, that 'the way in which professionals understand and perform their practice forms the basis for professional skill and its development'; secondly, that 'establishing a process of continual reflection and discussion' – that could be a consequence of transitioning to more individualised outcome-focused rather than time-based clinical practice[104] – 'would require substantial shifts in the current workplace culture of efficiency and performativity'. Critical reflection on practice may also be made more feasible through 'aspects of curriculum design that promote such achievement', as discussed further in Chapter 4.

Medical education

Learning systems review and development

Rationales for change: a recap

Major educational priorities from Australian,[100] Canadian,[101] US[102–106] and UK[107,108] reports were summarised in Chapter 3 along with some of the challenges of implementing changes. For these four countries, there appears to be consensus around a number of issues: the need for greater clarity of learning outcomes and more user-friendly curriculum syllabi or guidance, individualisation of learning, improved assessment tools and feedback, preventive medicine, along with better integration of interprofessionalism, technology, knowledge, science, humanities and clinical application, to name but a few. Most of these priorities are also congruent with the report *Health Professionals for a New Century: transforming education to strengthen health systems in an interdependent world.*[56]

Although arguments in favour of these changes are quite straightforward, they are perhaps not universally understood or welcomed. As discussed in earlier chapters, in the developed world many patients in the next few decades will have different personal and medical needs than those in the late twentieth and early twenty-first centuries, requiring different approaches in medical and social care. Changing medical conditions have had a knock-on effect on national budgets, as most funding is now consumed by long-term care. The most pressing and more immediate need is finding a better balance between hospital-based and local hospital and community care.

Funded largely through government coffers, professional regulatory bodies are accountable for overseeing that the preparation of the professionals match patient or client needs. Attached to universities, medical schools are responsible for delivering education and training programmes that meet expectations, as set down by the regulatory bodies. Educationally, this arrangement means the curricula on offer need to be more responsive to changes in healthcare needs, the organisation and delivery of care, and the shifting expectations, as emphasised in the recent GMC report *The State of Medical Education and Practice 2011*.[108]

Generally speaking, most healthcare curricula in use today are founded on late twentieth- or early twenty-first-century social, health and economic assumptions. While changes are ongoing, they tend to be related more to the biomedical sciences and clinical training within existing curriculum structures and expectations rather than the need to respond more effectively to actual population needs, which call for interprofessional or transprofessional practice, preventive and holistic medicine, practising in the community, self and peer assessment, or generally encouraging students and trainees to take responsibility for excellence in patient care. Placements and rotations and other learning structures that are in place tend to be inflexible, with few allowances for meeting individual learner needs. For example, noting that there 'is evidence of unacceptable and largely unexplained variations in the quality of care', the recent GMC report recommends inter alia that 'postgraduate training should be reviewed to ensure it is flexible enough to allow doctors to move between specialties'.[108]

The bottom line is that in terms of healthcare, and confirmed by various national reports, for example, the recent US report *Ensuring an Effective Physician Workforce for the United States: recommendations for reforming graduate medical education to meet the needs of the public*[104] by the Macy Foundation, and *The Lancet* Commission report on a global scale,[56] things need to be done radically differently, and these changes will no doubt influence the character, structure and scope of healthcare education in years to come.

Three approaches to planning and operating educational systems

While an oversimplification, but attempting to make several points that may interest readers, Figure 4.1 depicts three basic ways of operating any educational 'system' by reflecting on the system components in terms of input, process and output. The term 'input' is used to cover all aspects or elements that go into the system – syllabi, students, staff, resources and so forth. 'Process' refers to the learning environment and how students actually engage in learning, while 'output' is the overall outcome (skills, knowledge, personal development) of the learning experience, as confirmed by assessment results, grades, certification and graduate career destinations.

In Model 1, taking a rather elitist approach, *F* stands for a 'fixed' level of input, for example, ensuring that each incoming student has at least three 'A' star* levels as in the United Kingdom or a high grade point average in other systems – perhaps 3.5 or higher – used in the United States and China. When these students proceed through the system, and continue to be motivated, they will have a better than average chance of doing well in their studies and would likely do well in a rigid, prescribed or 'fixed' (F) curriculum. They would also demonstrate proficiency in their examinations and will have, as a result, better than average career prospects.

Model 2 does not 'fix' entry-level requirements and accepts variability (V) in terms of previous education and background with more students gaining acceptance with poorer grades than in Model 1. If the learning environment remains inflexible, that is, it does not allow for individual differences or takes into consideration individual needs, then the outcomes will also be predictably variable (V), and grades will be distributed as on a normal curve, with about 10%–20% gaining As and about 10%–15% failing. Most will likely end up with Cs – a rather mediocre and demotivating result for most! One of the issues with this scenario is that on failing, most students would have to start again even though they may have passed some modules, but the system – which rewards overall achievement – may not cater for this eventuality. The other question is whether the student will be pre-tested before beginning the next course to see where the gaps are in his or her learning.

Finally, in Model 3, we again accept variability (V) in terms of incoming students – grades, language, learning styles and so forth – but if we also then respond to individual differences (for example, readiness and time to learn, resources to match conceptual levels, personal circumstances (e.g. child care), extra tutorials

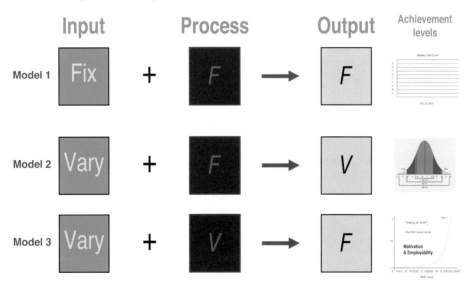

Personalising the learning experience!

FIGURE 4.1 Three modes of operating education systems[76]

and so forth), there is a greater likelihood that the students will achieve the outcomes, demonstrate personal satisfaction, higher motivation, self-confidence and better career prospects.

Many healthcare programmes – undergraduate and postgraduate – for a number of reasons, often outside the control of healthcare professionals (e.g. demand exceeding supply) do not always encourage meeting the highest standards or 'excellence' in patient care and presently apply Models 1 and 2 usually with good outcomes for students engaged in Model 1 learning environments (i.e. high entry requirements) but variable outcomes for those in Model 2 contexts, which may also explain the variability in patient care, as outlined in the GMC[108] and other reports.

A key to improving student and trainee performance may lie with increasingly adopting Model 3 in relation to healthcare education and training – beginning with identification of actual population needs and the specification of meaningful competencies and student/trainee-friendly learning outcomes and ensuring the students or trainees have the opportunity to be engaged in appropriate clinical contexts and collaborative learning experiences.

Regardless of the model, all healthcare training providers have the responsibility for the overview of academic standards and quality assurance and enhancement processes and in the development of policy and practice in relation to them. Quality assurance is essentially a process that ensures that the training is 'fit for purpose' and ensures that the training meets internal and external standards (for example, the GMC in the United Kingdom). In the past decade there has been an increasing emphasis on institutional and programme self-reviews based on multiple feedback mechanisms, in particular valuing the student or trainee 'voice', especially since a central aim of all quality processes is to ensure that employees take full responsibility for their actions. As Henry Ford is reported to have said, quality means 'doing it right when no one is looking'. While the three models share these aims and approaches, Model 3, as discussed further in this chapter, may necessitate applying additional quality metrics and paying more attention to the learning experience of 'individual' learners in relation to learning outcomes, teaching and learning methods, modes of delivery, assessments, learning environments and personal support. These aspects would likely benefit from the use of individualised or personalised learning contracts or agreements worked out by the educational mentor or supervisor and the trainee. In addition, more emphasis may need to be placed on patient and peer feedback as well as personal reflection on practice and interactions. Collectively, in Model 3 learning contexts, this information should feed into quality enhancement activities not only to ensure quality control processes are meeting specified standards but also to optimise creativity, innovation and individuality.

Reconceptualising healthcare education and training

Figure 4.2 compares the traditional 'educational' curriculum model that 'emphasises memorisation and recall'[144] to the competency-based model. And, rather than the existing curriculum or available texts driving learning leading to educational objectives, the competency-based approach focuses on health and health system needs and the competency expectations of graduates (i.e. what the graduate has to be able to do or demonstrate in the work environment) accompanied by authentic standards.

In terms of healthcare the competency-based approach would first need 'to specify the health problems to be addressed, the living and health contexts in which they occur, societal trends and identify the requisite competencies required of graduates for health-system performance, tailor the curriculum to achieve competencies, and assess achievements and shortfalls'.

Gruppen, Mangrulkar, and Kaolars, authors of *The Lancet*-commissioned paper *Competency-Based Education in the Health professions: implications for improving global health*,[145] cite Albanese *et al.*,[146] who identify four key characteristics that define a competency:

1. A competency focuses on the performance or the end product or goal-state of instruction.
2. A competency reflects expectations that are external to the immediate institutional programme.

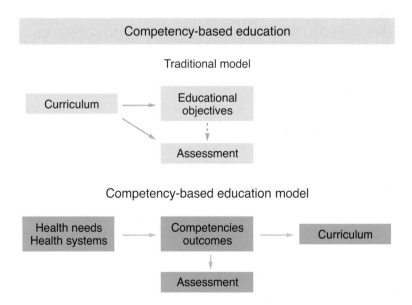

FIGURE 4.2 *The Lancet* report: transforming twentieth-century healthcare curricula[56]

3. A competency is expressible in terms of measurable behaviour.
4. A competency informs learners as well as other stakeholders about what is expected of them.

If these criteria were applied rigorously to healthcare training, then 'the mismatch between competencies to patient and population needs', identified in *The Lancet* report,[56] it is argued, could be largely resolved, and more doctors, nurses and other health/social care professionals would be enabled to care for their patients with improved skills, knowledge and professional formation.

Further, Gruppen, Mangrulkar, and Kaolars[145] conclude that '[t]raditional education tends to focus on what and how learners are taught and less so on whether or not they can use their learning to solve problems, perform procedures, communicate effectively, or make good clinical decisions.' And '[b]y emphasising the results of education rather than its processes, CBE [competency-based education] provides a significant, even dramatic shift in what educators and policy-makers look for in judging the effectiveness of educational programs.' According to the authors, '[t]he curriculum, or what is to be learned, is at the heart of all educational models. It is the genesis or origin of the curriculum that differentiates traditional models from CBE.' They continue:

> Historically, the professions themselves have set requirements that serve to determine who can obtain membership based on completion of curricula that they determine. While often positioning themselves to serve the public good, there is also a tendency to serve the needs of their own professions and members. Curricula often become anchored to historical legacies that codify the traditions, priorities, and values of the faculty in that profession. Over time, the curricula are modified with new information. Typically, this is additive with less attention to the removal of elements that are less pertinent to current practice. Often, it is the expansion of new scientific knowledge that drives the curriculum, at the expense of a focus on the implementation of what is already known to be of benefit.

In addition, the authors observe that '[a]lthough there has been a greater focus on the need for learning objectives in the health professions, it is not uncommon for schools to "retrofit" the objectives to reflect what the faculty desire to teach. In this sense, the curriculum drives the objectives rather than the desired learning objectives driving the curriculum. This framework then results in a system of assessment that is again based on the mastery of a curriculum that may be detached from the needs of society.'[145]

The crucial point here is that it is time for change: we need to match training competencies of all healthcare professionals to actual population needs – now and project five to ten years from now and involve all key stakeholders – medical practitioners, allied health professionals, trainees, lay persons – … in deciding and prioritising competencies.

A possible dilemma facing regulatory professional bodies across the globe, including the Royal Colleges in the United Kingdom, and medical educators generally, may be how to make radical changes, articulated in *The Lancet* and other reports, while having to continue with existing structures and arrangements. Professor Samuel Thier,[147] professor emeritus of medicine and health policy at Harvard Medical School, at the launch of *The Lancet* Commission report, emphasised:

> First and foremost, the need for existing educational programs will not stop while we are innovating. Thus any innovation must assume that while moving from idea to execution there remains an acceptable level of functioning. The greater the change produced by innovation, the more critical it is to assure a safe, effective transition period. This concern may dictate the use of pilot programs and limit the number of participants to manageable size.

It is well known that reconceptualising and redesigning curricula is resource intensive and that developments take time, with funding already stretched to capacity in most countries. While these issues will need to be tackled locally, one consideration for planners could be to bring together leaders from health and social care, including patient and client representatives, to map out a comprehensive strategic framework for enacting transformative curriculum change – a 'master' blueprint that could drive changes in specific health and social care curricula forward, embracing key features: competency-based, including identifying common inter/trans-professional competencies (e.g. anatomy, physiology, infection control, gerontology, patient safety in clinical practice, health promotion and public health); matching learning outcomes to population needs; rebalancing community and hospital care; authentic assessments; effective and user-friendly syllabi; and optimising technology-mediated resources.

To these ends, it is suggested that the *CIIC* framework (Figure 4.3), which identifies four fundamental cornerstones of future curriculum development – **C**ompetencies, **I**ntegration, **I**nter/trans-professionalism and **C**reativity – could be facilitative in redesigning healthcare curricula. The main components could also lead to the development of new metrics to ensure programmes are up to date and are quality assured in terms of levels of integration and inter/trans-professionalism, and that they are delivered creatively and flexibly in terms of resources, time and location – especially taking advantage of mediated learning and technology.

- *Competencies*: a major challenge for planners is how to incorporate all the different competencies, new domains of knowledge and emergent disciplines into the curriculum in order to produce a more complete healthcare worker – one that meets the needs of individuals and populations.

● *Integration*: another significant issue emerging from the competency umbrella is how best to structure the curriculum and reconcile knowledge requirements and clinical experience, science and the humanities, hospital and community care as well as health and social care.

● *Inter/trans-professionalism*: as outlined earlier, this needs to become a top priority in health and social care, encouraging, for example, more common (clinical and non-clinical) learning with allied health and social care professions.

● *Creativity*: there are many areas where new ways of thinking to enhance the learning experience could apply – assessment, technology, rotations. This is an issue also highlighted in Britain by Professor Sir Peter Rubin, chair of the GMC, as '[i]ntensive, but unsupervised experience is not a substitute for properly supervised training, delivered by consultants who have the time to do it'.[148]

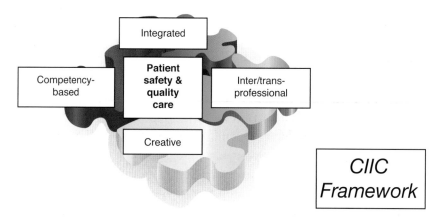

FIGURE 4.3 Proposed core healthcare curriculum design framework

Mapping population health and competency needs using the *DACUM* process

The authors of *The Lancet*-commissioned report[56] see a 'potentially transformative use of competencies'. They could, for example:

> serve as an objective basis for classification of the various health professions, instead of the present arbitrary borders, which are indicative of the relative success of different occupational groups in mobilisation of the powers of the State to award credentials specifically to establish monopolies of practice. Attainment of specific competencies, not time or academic turf protection,

must be the defining feature of the education and evaluation of future health professionals.

Approaching curricula in this way could be very useful in supporting both local and large-scale curriculum development projects, in particular when emerging professions or occupations are scrutinised or when existing professions or occupations need to undergo major refocusing. The current WHO project *Increasing Access to Health Workers in Remote and Rural Areas through Improved Retention*[149] may be an example of both cases. The rationales for the project is summarised succinctly by the director-general of WHO, Dr Margaret Chan:

> Half the world's people currently live in rural and remote areas. The problem is that most health workers live and work in cities. This imbalance is common to almost all countries and poses a major challenge to the nationwide provision of health services. Its impact, however, is most severe in low-income countries. There are two reasons for this. One is that many of the countries already suffer from acute shortages of health workers – in all areas. The other is that the proportion of the population living in rural regions tends to be in poorer countries than in rich ones.

The WHO expert panel, co-chaired by Dr Manuel Dayrit, former Secretary of Health (Minister) of the Philippines, and now Director of Human Resources at WHO, and Professor Charles Normand, an economist and Edward Kennedy Professor of Health Policy and Management at the University of Ireland, identified a number of strategies 'to help countries encourage health workers to live and work in remote and rural areas'. Recommendations fell into four main categories: (1) educational, (2) regulatory, (3) financial and (4) personal/professional. A key recommendation is to 'revise undergraduate and postgraduate curricula to include health topics so as to enhance the competencies of health professionals working in rural areas, and thereby increase their job satisfaction and retention'.

There are a number of advantages to proceeding down the competency curriculum development route, including 'laddering' within and across professions, planning of 'community experiences clinical rotations' and designing 'continuing education and professional development programmes that meet the needs of rural health workers and that are accessible from where they live and work, so as to support their retention.'[149] In addition, *The Lancet* Commission report[56] notes:

> Once educators focus on professional competencies, new opportunities emerge for a more imaginative design of health systems. Roles and compensation can be better aligned. Traditional boundaries between professions can be reduced. The pervasive trend towards credential creep between professions

– i.e. the trend whereby the credentials required for a specific position are increasing – can be challenged.

An innovative technique that has been proven to effectively and efficiently identify competencies and develop multidisciplinary frameworks, pioneered in Canada, is called *DACUM*, an acronym that stands for **D**esigning **A** Curricul**UM**.[150,151]

Four key assumptions underpin the process:
1. Experts can define and describe their roles more accurately than anyone else.
2. Any profession or occupation can be effectively described in terms of the competencies that successful professionals perform.
3. All professions and occupations demand certain knowledge, skills and attitudes from employees.
4. Roles develop over time and need to adapt to changing environments.

Curriculum mapping is simply a process that ensures that students, trainees and supervisors know where they are going, why they are going there, and what

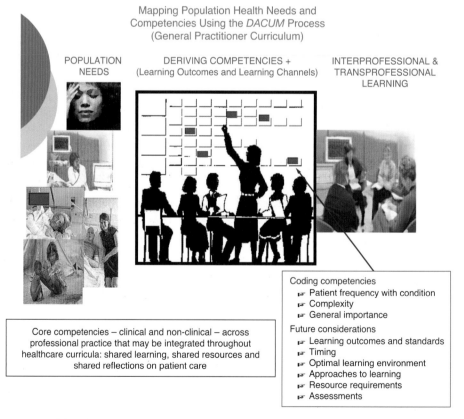

FIGURE 4.4 Mapping competencies using the *DACUM* process

is required of them to get there. *DACUM* is primarily concerned with the first two questions and is a facilitated curriculum mapping or storyboarding process (Figure 4.4), which normally takes 2–3 days to complete and can involve about 15–20 expert practitioners – from early, mid, and late career – drawn carefully from a cross-section of professional fields. With regard to potential healthcare analyses using DACUM, contributors would likely include a mix of doctors, nurses, midwives, pharmacists, radiologists and social workers, to name just a few.

As shown in Figure 4.4, the main reason for coming together is to discuss, debate, define and agree core and interdependent competencies[56,144] that are necessary (e.g. in the case of healthcare). The resultant documentation or 'blueprint' – normally a chart or profile providing a summary of major areas and intermediate areas of competencies – can then be validated or triangulated through additional survey research involving other practitioners, nationally or globally.

Benefits of applying *DACUM* in healthcare curricula

While there are other methods for identifying competencies or doing a 'front-end analysis', as the process is frequently called (e.g. surveys, interviews, existing documentation), the *DACUM* process is one of the few methods that engages stakeholders (local, national, international) directly, builds relationships understanding and commitment, helps to raise awareness of key issues and begins the journey for further planning and decision-making. While it can take months to gather data from surveys and interviews, and relying on texts published several years previously can be risky, the *DACUM* process can take only a few days to identify key competencies and compile highly relevant and timely information to guide further instructional development.

Another strength of the approach is that it can promote discussion of transdisciplinary medical education needs, where competencies are centred on issues, problems, needs or themes. These needs then form the basis of the learning outcomes, applied to a particular programme. Moreover, participants who are involved in the process become, in a sense, leaders or 'seed carriers' or catalysts for change. Their background and experience also enables them to further progress the curriculum design or redesign.

The approach is also useful in developing career ladders and lattices, as shown in Figure 4.5, and advocated by the US Department of Labor's Competency Model Clearinghouse.[152] Whereas 'career ladders display only vertical movement between jobs, career lattices contain both vertical and lateral movement between jobs and may reflect more closely the career paths of today's work environment'.

For example, the career lattice in Figure 4.5 enables healthcare professionals

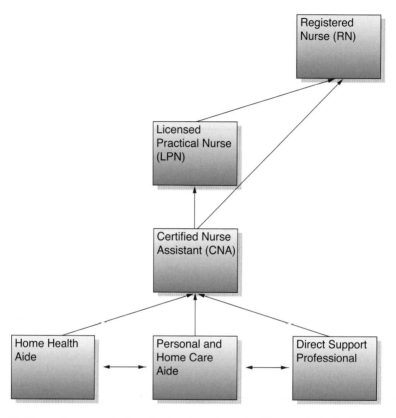

FIGURE 4.5 Example career lattice for the long-term healthcare industry[152]

to move in several directions rather than just upward. The arrows leading from Home Health Aide to Certified Nurse Assistant (CNA) to Licensed Practical Nurse (LPN) to Registered Nurse (RN) portray vertical movement between jobs. The arrows between Home Health Aide, Personal and Home Care Aide, and Direct Support Professional portray lateral movement between jobs.

In terms of healthcare education and training, *DACUM* has the potential to provide an effective, fast and economical means for the development of new outcomes-based programmes or to help ensure that existing programmes/courses meet present and future expectations, benefiting professional regulatory bodies, clinicians, students or trainees.

Case examples

Learning systems implementation

The University of the Philippines Manila School of Health Science: 'where health workers are trained to stay and serve'[153]

The laddering approach, discussed in the previous chapter, is used at the University of the Philippines (UP) Manila School of Health Science (SHS), which was 'established by UP in response to the brain drain and maldistribution of health manpower prevailing in the country in the 1970s'.[153] Another major factor in the 1970s was that UP was concerned that 'its programs in the health sciences were breeding a generation of individualistic, self-centered, and grade-conscious students who did not care whether their education would help them serve the country'. Recognising that a major change was necessary, an Extraordinary Curriculum Committee of the UP College of Medicine 'was tasked to design a medical curriculum that would train graduates who are scientifically disciplined, medically competent, and more importantly, socially conscious, community-oriented, and firmly committed to serve the people'.

What makes this programme unique is that 'the community is an essential partner in carrying out the programme, from the recruitment of SHS scholars to the employment of SHS graduates. Scholars at the SHS are recruited from and endorsed by depressed communities in the country in dire need of health workers.' On admission to the programme, 'the scholar enters into a social contract with the community and pledges to return to the latter to render service as a health worker upon completion of his/her training. The community in turn pledges a measure of support for this scholar while he or she is at the school and during service leaves, which refers to service in one's community of origin after completing a level in the curriculum.'

Another aspect that distinguishes the programme from others is the stepladder curriculum, which is 'an innovative community-based and competency-based programme that integrates the training of barangay health workers (BHW[s]), midwives, nurses and physicians in a single, sequential, and continuous curriculum'. Other innovative features, as shown in Figure 5.1, include:

> multiple levels of entry and exit, enabling the scholar to exit at any level and return to serve the community with the competence of the level he or she has attained. Hence, one may exit as a BHW, midwife, nurse, or physician. The scholar may be readmitted directly to the next level after completion of the service leave or after having rendered a longer period of service in the community through employment or voluntary service. After serving the community, should there be a need for a health worker with more advanced knowledge and skills, the scholar may be admitted to the next level of the curriculum. For each level, the student develops competencies in order to fulfill five major roles: (1) health care provider, (2) community mobilizer and organizer, (3) health service manager, (4) trainer/educator, and (5) researcher.

The entry point into the curriculum is the Certificate of Barangay Health Work, which is completed in one quarter or 11 weeks. Those who complete the certificate programme go back to their places of origin to render service leave. Scholars who return and study for six more quarters (18 months) graduate with a Certificate in Community Health Work.

University of the Philippines School of Health Sciences, Leyte[153]
Fast facts

Created: 1976

Location: Tacloban City, Leyte Island, the Philippines

Curriculum: 5-year MD curriculum that students in underserved areas enter upon the completion of a single, integrated, sequential, and continuous curriculum that begins with community-health worker training (Midwifes) and practice, Mid-wifery training and practice, then a BA in nursing. The MD program alternates didactics, community work and clinical work. Graduates then complete National Physicians Licensure Exams.

Mission

Develop outstanding and committed health professionals who will stay and serve in the Philippines through excellent community-based, competency based, community oriented education directed towards service in depressed and underserved areas of the country.

Strategies

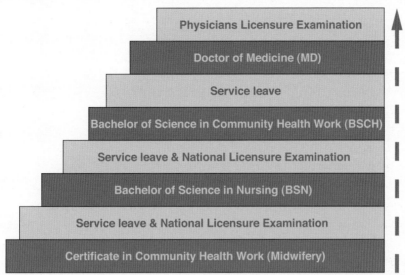

Physicians Licensure Examination

Doctor of Medicine (MD)

Service leave

Bachelor of Science in Community Health Work (BSCH)

Service leave & National Licensure Examination

Bachelor of Science in Nursing (BSN)

Service leave & National Licensure Examination

Certificate in Community Health Work (Midwifery)

FIGURE 5.1 Stepladder curriculum: community and competency-based

Certification in Community Health Work (7 Q = 21 months)
BS Nursing (add 5 Q =15 months)
Doctor of Medicine (add 20 Q = 5 years)

Service leave

A period in-between program levels for when students are required to return
to their sponsoring communities to render health and community development
services for an indefinite period or a minimum of three months. This enables
scholars to learn and serve at the same time within the context of their home
communities.

Multiple entry and exit mechanisms

- Students may exit from any level of the curriculum and return to the
  community as a functional health worker
- After a period of serving the community, a graduate can be readmitted to the
  next level of the curriculum subject to community need and endorsement

Partnership with linked agencies and communities in the development of Health Human Resources

- Involvement of DOH,[a] DILG[b] and LGUs[c] in recruitment of scholars
- Endorsement is required for scholar's admission and progress to higher levels

- University, linked agencies and LGUs share the responsibility of providing financial support for scholars
- Shared supervision of the students during service leave between the school, linked agencies and community
- Lecturers are sourced primarily from the DOH.

Democratized admission
- Students don't take UPCAT[d]
- Students are admitted on the basis of community need rather than past academic performance
- Qualitative grading system of 'Passed' (P) and 'Needs Tutorial' (NT) ensures development of required competencies rather than competing for grades.

Return service requirement
- Sponsoring communities are committed to employ their scholars after graduation
- Scholars are required a return service obligation of 2 years service for every year of study which ensures the availability of health workers especially in underserved areas.

Outcomes and contributions
Local
- has recruited close to three thousand (3,000) scholars from 73 provinces all over the Philippines
- Graduated midwives, nurses and doctors, 85% of whom are still serving in depressed and underserved areas of the Philippines
- Passing rates in National Examinations
  —Midwifery – 97–100%, with examinees consistently in the top ten
  —Nursing – 86–95% also with top ten examinees
  —MD – has licensed more than 75% of its graduates
- Pioneer and leader of ladderized curriculum, community-based and competency-based education in the Philippines
- Venue for training of health human resources of special groups as the ARMM,[e] Indigenous People and other community-based organizations
- Acclaimed and evaluated nationally as an effective strategy to fill in the need for Health Human Resource in underserved areas of the country
- Influenced the integration and restructuring of the health care delivery system in the Philippines

- Community empowerment through educational opportunities for scholars from disadvantaged areas.

International

- Principal field experience for Health for All policy and the PHC[f] policy of the Philippines and the WHO-Western Pacific Region
- Training venue for JICA[g] Trainings for Prospective PHC workers now fielded in 26 developing countries
- Hosted various international study visits.

Notes: [a]Department of Health; [b]Department of the Interior and Local Government; [c]local government units; [d]UP College Admission Test; [e]Autonomous Region of Muslim Mindanao; [f]primary health care; [g]Japan International Cooperation Agency.

To date, the programme has graduated 2860 students, of whom 126 (4.4%) became medical doctors and fewer than 10% have gone abroad. Benefits of the community-based approach being taken to the training of healthcare professionals include 'less attrition and waste of resources as a scholar may exit at any level of the curriculum and become a functional health worker in the health care system'. Further, '[t]he multiple entry and exit mechanism allows for the progressive, unified, and continuous development of competencies of a specific health worker needed by the community'.

Moreover, proceeding 'through the ladder promotes team spirit among health workers and makes them better appreciate their role as multi-skilled health professionals who would meet the needs of the country's rural poor'.[153]

However, according to the writer Josie Lydia J Siega-Sur, associate professor and dean at the University of the Philippines Manila School of Health Sciences, the main benefit is that 'the step-ladder approach cultivates the culture of service to the country'.[154]

From competencies to learning outcomes

Generally speaking, competencies refer to knowledge, skills and attitudes expected in a professional or vocational role. These are then cast into learning goals (broad statements of intent) and learning outcomes (more specific statements of intent) that are essentially the steps to achieving the competencies. Ideally, trainees should encounter, in a graduated way, 'increasingly clinical challenges and decreasing supervisory intervention' to ensure the safety of patients and to enable accurate assessment of their capabilities'.[102]

Formulating learning outcomes that matter and motivate[155] is crucial to designing or redesigning a learning system that meets the needs of learners and societal expectations and that could respond to issues identified in recent reports on medical education. Several professions have applied SMART criteria to ensure their outcomes are of a high standard and are found to be helpful to the students and trainees.[156]

> **S – Specific**: to tell learners or a team exactly what is expected, why it is important, who is involved, where it is going to happen and which attributes are important.
>
> **M – Measurable**: to provide concrete criteria for measuring progress toward the attainment of the outcome, including knowledge, skill and professional formation/attitudinal aspects.
>
> **A – Attainable**: to ensure that the learning outcomes are realistic and achievable in the time available – that is, neither out of reach nor below standard performance, as these may be considered meaningless.
>
> **R – Realistic**: to ensure that the students/trainees are able to progressively study and care for patients from a cross-section of conditions or illnesses that actually represent their patients when they start to practise on completion and to set the bar high enough for a satisfying achievement – not too high, not too low!
>
> **T – Timebound**: to specify a timeframe as commitment to a deadline helps learners or a team focus their efforts on completion of the learning outcome or prevent goals from being overtaken by the day-to-day crises that invariably arise in patient care situations.

On a more whimsical, but salient note, the importance of knowing one's destination is made clear in the encounter between Alice and the Cheshire cat in *Alice's Adventures in Wonderland*: 'Which road do I take?' asks Alice. The cat replies, 'Where do you want to go?' 'I don't know,' Alice answers. 'Then,' says the cat, 'it doesn't matter. If you don't know where you are going, any road will get you there.' Of course, the problem in healthcare education is that without well-defined competencies and learning outcomes there is a high probability of a mismatch between health system and patient needs and what students and trainees learn. In addition, not knowing specifically what is expected of the healthcare professional can lead to confusion, unsafe practice, inefficiency and compromise the quality of patient care.[56,146]

Another difficulty with existing learning outcomes in healthcare education is that often students and trainees are faced with comprehensive lists of what needs to be learned – knowledge, skills, professionalism – but they have difficulty deciding on priorities and many find it even more demanding to contextualise the outcomes within the clinical environments. Surely not everything is of equal importance. Given the variability of training environments, the question arises whether the healthcare training experience should be determined mostly by the availability of patients or by a curriculum that ensures balance and depth across healthcare practice through more deliberate, intentional longitudinal placements or rotations.[102] Rather than moving through progressive development stages, the learning experience for many healthcare students can often feel disorganised or overwhelming, especially when coupled with the tension between service and training requirements. One consequence is that few students or trainees or supervisors for that matter appear to have enough time to pay sufficient attention to the documentation that is made available to them.

A possible solution to this issue is to find ways of better integrating curriculum guidance within the training schemes and placing more responsibility on students or trainees to monitor their work performance, including through peer review and ideally patient feedback.

A case study in curriculum mapping of core medicine

In a curriculum-mapping project, sponsored by the UK Kent, Surrey and Sussex Postgraduate Deanery, several consultant education advisers and key staff members from a large Trust tried to broach this problem by developing a 'Curriculum in Practice' core medical training framework.

Basing their approach on the comprehensive *Generic Curriculum for the Medical Specialties*[157] and the *Specialty Training Framework for Core Medical Training*,[158] both documents prepared by the Royal College of Physicians (RCP), consultants and trainees were asked to participate in a curriculum-mapping project. Through face-to-face interviews and online feedback, the exercise – a modified *DACUM* approach – was essentially a 'situation analysis … to recognise the complex realities of medical practice', in particular, 'as it exists in the given context on the ground'.[159] Those interviewed were asked to reflect on the trainee experience from induction to near completion of the core curriculum and to find out the extent to which the local curriculum aligned with the national curriculum. It also involved prioritising and coding the RCP competencies in terms of frequency of patients seen, level of complexity involved in diagnoses and treatment and general importance of the competency in the general scheme of things. Following the RCP curriculum, competencies had been grouped under five categories: (1) generic, (2) symptom-based, (3) system-based, (4) investigation and (5) procedural. In addition, consultants were asked about available learning opportunities at three hospitals.

Their collective feedback informed the curriculum section in the trainee handbook, outlining the main learning outcome for each competency category (*see* Figure 5.2), along with specific competencies. The competency framework could be helpful in the first interview with their educational supervisor, where discussions focus on achieving the competencies in the 2-year timeframe. Trainees are also encouraged to use the pro forma to monitor their progress at intervals of 8 or 9, 16 and 22 or 23 months, using a 5-point proficiency scale (1 = low experience; 3 = moderate experience; 5 = high experience) against the standards set out in the Core Medical Training *Annual Review of Competence Progression Decision Aid Standards* (ARCP).

II. Symptom-based Competencies

Emergency Presentations

At the end of CMT 2, you should be able to assess a patient presenting with the condition, produce a valid differential diagnosis, investigate appropriately, formulate and implement a management plan when presented with the following conditions.

As evidenced in your e-portfolio (ACAT[1]/CbD[2]/mini-CEX[3]):
- **at month 8 or 9** you are expected to demonstrate **some experience of all.**
- **at month 16** you are expected to be **competent in all.**
- **at month 22 or 23** you are expected to be **competent in all.**

[1] ACAT = Acute Care Assessment Tool

[2] CbD = Case-based Discussion

[3] Mini-CEX = Mini Clinical Evaluation Exercise

Competency	Learning Opportunities	Reference *CMTF*	8/9 M PL	16 M PL	22/23 M PL
1. Cardio-Respiratory Arrest	OC/FTP	p. 43			
2. Shocked Patient	WW/OC	p. 43			
3. Unconscious Patient	WW/OC	p. 44			
4. Anaphylaxis	FTP/SDL/WW	p. 45			

Column 1: Competencies 1 and 2 were given a high priority by the consultants and trainees.

Column 2: Identifies learning opportunities (e.g. OC = on call; FTP = formal teaching; WW = Ward Work; SDL= self-directed learning) etc.

Column 3: Cross-references competencies to learning outcomes in Core Medical Training Framework[80]

Column 4: PL – Proficiency Level – Self-assessments at 8/9, 16, 22/23 month intervals.

FIGURE 5.2 Example of a proposed core medical training 'curriculum in practice' handbook excerpt

The self-assessments are meant to support reflections on their training and could also be helpful in meetings with their educational supervisors, who may provide further career guidance or support in preparation for the *Annual Review of Competence Progression Decision Aid Standards*. Moreover, each competency was cross-referenced to the more detailed learning outcomes specified in the RCP *Specialty Training Framework for Core Medical Training*, and in future could also be linked to resources. It remains to be seen whether such an approach will be helpful in creating awareness of expectations and closing the gap between curriculum documentation and making best use of it.

Adapting healthcare curricula to the twenty-first century

In adapting or redesigning healthcare curricula for the twenty-first century, we need to be mindful of specifying and integrating the various dimensions previously identified, and absent in most medical curricula – balancing uniprofessional and clinical practice in community settings, for example. These changes may necessitate reviewing entire curricula to provide a better balance and cohesion, (for example, with regard to curative and preventive medicine, inter/trans-professional learning, clinical practice in local or community settings). Consistent with Learning Systems Design principles, the development of curricula may be facilitated by sequentially asking the following questions:

- What are learners expected to do or demonstrate in relation to the outcomes that they could not do beforehand?
- How well prepared are they in relation to the expected aims and outcomes?
- What are the most realistic, feasible and cost-effective approaches to delivering the course or unit?
- How will learners and tutors know that the students' level of proficiency – knowledge, skills, attitudes – is at, or better still beyond, a minimum standard of performance?
- Overall, how will the learning environment and experiences support achieving the outcomes?

Learning outcome components[155,156]

Four additional dimensions should be considered when writing learning outcomes:

1. As reflected by the expected competence (i.e. choice of action verb), they need to be written at *different levels of difficulty* to reflect actual performance

levels. As Table 5.1 shows, being able to 'label a diagram' is a lot easier than being able to 'propose an alternative diagnosis'. Over the years taxonomies have been developed for each domain (*see* point #4 in this list) to guide developers.[156]

2. They should indicate a *minimum standard of performance* – in terms of quality, quantity or time, or a combination of these.

3. They should specify the *condition or circumstances* under which the performance is carried out.

4. They should be written in *three main domains*: Knowledge (Cognitive), Skills (Psychomotor) and Professional Formation (Affective), as they are in the RCP *Core Medical Specialty Training Framework.*

TABLE 5.1 Examples of learning outcomes in medical education[154]

Type	Conditions	Outcomes	Standards
Knowledge	On a simplified diagram of the body	**Label** vital organs of each system of the body	All placed correctly
Knowledge	Provided a case study diagnosis	**Predict** consequences (on other systems) of the malfunctioning of a given body system	Making at least 3 predictions per case
Knowledge	Without access to diagnostic equipment or references	**Propose** an alternative diagnosis	Citing at least two items of evidence which refute the diagnosis
Skill	Given a new patient to clerk	**Perform** a complete physical examination	Completing all steps as set out in the clinical assessment manual.
Professional formation	In weekly multidisciplinary patient review meetings	**Volunteer** to be critically evaluated by others	Accepting feedback in a positive fashion as evidenced by …

Learning systems design: ensuring patient safety and learning effectiveness

Alarmed by an article that suggested hospital staff shortages 'cause 500 deaths a year', Sir Roy Thompson,[160] president of the UK Royal College of Physicians, noted that 'too few junior doctors are caring for too many patients overnight and at the weekend'. Concerned with patient safety and quality care, he noted further that '[p]atients who are admitted to hospital in the evening and at the weekend risk receiving sub-standard care' and that '[d]espite the best efforts of consultants who work above their contracted hours, patients are not getting sufficient input to their care from senior doctors during these periods'. With respect to medical education, he observes that '[t]he supervision and training of junior doctors is also adversely affected by a lack of senior input during these periods. More doctors are required to provide this high level service.' He then calls for 'an urgent need to review workforce patterns in hospitals to ensure that medical in-patients receive direct input from consultant physicians on every day of the week'. As this situation points out, there is an urgent need to tackle healthcare improvements on many fronts – matching patient needs to treatments and support as well as structuring the care so that there is a consistent and reliable workforce available to the patients in the first place. Systematic planning must replace what seem to be ad hoc arrangements when it comes to much patient care. From these situations, we may conclude that the more complex the clinical environment, the greater the need for managing the care 24/7. Similar problems are occurring in other health systems. For example, in the United States, Dr James Battles,[161] a senior service fellow for patient safety at the Agency for Healthcare Research and Quality, reminds us that '[a]ll too often we have relied on training as the only interventions for patient safety without examining other alternatives or realising that, in some cases, the training systems themselves are part of the problem'. Further, he advises that '[o]ne way to ensure safety by design is to apply established design principles to education and training' and recommends the use of instructional systems design principles. Instructional systems design, preferably called 'Learning Systems Design', is 'a systematic method of development of education and training programs for improved learner performance and involves five integrated steps: Analysis, Development, Design, Implementation, and Evaluation (ADDIE).' He concludes that 'the ADDIE approach can eliminate or prevent education and training from being a contributing factor of health associated injury or harm, and can also be effective in preventing injury or harm.

Frequently placed 'at the sharp end', he posits, 'trainees, whether nursing or medical students, graduate medical trainees, pharmacists, or allied health professions students, errors in one part of the system place other components at significant risk'. While 'in many error critical situations … the learning process takes place in a protected environment such as a simulator to minimize the risk to the public … this is not always the case in health care, especially in teaching hospitals and clinics where trainees deliver a significant level of care to patients'. His main message – based on over 25 years' experience – is 'that education and training activities must be carefully designed in order to be effective, and that using the ADDIE approach is one way by which we can make health care safer by design'.

Figure 5.3 applies ADDIE principles to the design of medical education and training programmes, courses or placements and identifies six key stages of formulating performance-driven curricula, including the Analysis Stage, including the identification of competencies and learning outcomes discussed earlier. When students or trainees do not succeed at any level in their curriculum, problems can usually be traced back to one or more of these development and implementation phases. For example, it is possible that the competencies and learning outcomes were set at too high a level or were not comprehensive or sharp enough to the students or trainees or that assumptions about the incoming students or trainees were inaccurate or unrealistic. Perhaps many had not taken a course in biology or had not worked interprofessionally. Equally the learning environment may have been unsuitable in supporting the anticipated outcomes – too many episodic encounters and not a wide enough range of patient conditions and possibly the assessments did not reflect the outcomes, did not provide enough formative practice or feedback was sparse or non-existent. In any case, the last stage is one where these types of questions need to be raised for each student or trainee along with the entire cohort. At this point feedback to the students and trainees is very important to detail strengths and weaknesses of the curriculum, and, most important, what has been or will be done about issues or problems by the course team.

Increasingly, medical educators are also reminded to raise awareness about issues or concerns that stem from the 'hidden' curriculum, whereby what students

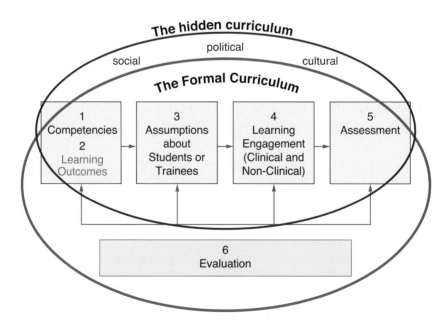

FIGURE 5.3 Learning systems design: ensuring patient safety and learning effectiveness[155]

or trainees learn is much more than the sum total of the curriculum. Becoming a doctor also needs to be understood as a socialisation process which is strongly influenced by social, political and cultural factors.[162,163] As Dr Tom Dolphin of the British Medical Association's junior doctors committee points out, '[b]eing a doctor in Britain requires much more than just clinical expertise. It is also important to have highly developed communication skills, knowledge of UK medical ethics and culture, and an understanding of how the NHS works.'[164] The forthcoming changes in health and social care may be a prime area for open debate and discussion.

An example of creating an interprofessional, innovative and engaging learning environment

The Competency, Integration, Interprofessional and Creative framework, suggested as a cornerstone for curriculum design in Chapter 4, emphasises the importance of striving to provide creative learning experiences that go beyond 'traditional lecturing and note-taking, certified by periodic examinations'.[165]

This traditional approach to teaching has been of long-standing concern, some may say since the thirteenth or fourteenth centuries, and certainly does not reflect the twenty-first-century *learner*, who, aside from school or college, has grown up in a multi-mediated world, where, unlike many present-day curricula, he or she needs to interact with a world that demands instant access to information and which is highly unpredictable, far removed from the certainties of large group lectures and multiple-choice examinations.

In the United States, the Boyer Commission,[165] sponsored by the Carnegie Foundation for the Advancement of Teaching, was also highly critical of undergraduate teaching at universities, advocating a model of teaching where students have 'opportunities to learn through inquiry rather than simple transmission of knowledge'. That was over 14 years ago, yet the traditional model of teaching persists to this day in classrooms and lecture theatres across the globe. Seen historically, it was 'created for a time when books were scarce and costly; lecturing to large audiences of students was an efficient means of creating several compendia of learning where only one existed before'. According to the Commission, '[t]he delivery system persisted into the present largely because it was familiar, easy, and required no imagination' and 'the experience of most undergraduates at most research universities is that of receiving what is served out to them. In one course after another they listen, transcribe, absorb, and repeat essentially as undergraduates have done for centuries'.

While in many institutions the Boyer Commission's observations are still valid, in many countries things are changing.[166] However, according to *The*

Lancet Commission, '[e]ducational institutions must now be re-engineered to adapt to this transformation; otherwise they risk becoming obsolete'. Further, the Commission makes clear that 'the use of IT [information technology] might be the most important driver in transformative learning – one of the guiding notions' of their report. From their perspective 'IT-empowered learning is already a reality for the younger generation in most countries, and in many cases, the uptake of new digital technologies has been faster and more widespread in poor rather than in rich countries'.[56]

Imaginative teaching does not of course always have to be rooted in IT but can activate learning channels that draw on 'didactic faculty lectures, small student learning groups, team-based education'[56] (to name but a few approaches), as is the case with Professor Claudia Diaz's anatomy classes at James Cook University in Australia![167]

Here Professor Diaz's main aim is 'to provide a nurturing and stimulating environment for students' that will also make learning 'enjoyable'. Being an enthusiastic teacher, Professor Diaz, in her own words, is on an important mission 'to change the historical views regarding the teaching and learning of anatomy'. She is a realist, fully recognising the inherent and contextual challenges of learning anatomy, such as the difficulty of 'learning new concepts and complex terminologies' with students 'finding their efforts on memorising "lists" of names in typical surface-learning approaches' both 'dull and labour intensive'.

Other pressures at Australian universities have led to reducing contact hours for anatomy. Classes are large and incoming health science students are very diverse in terms of 'entry level, prior experience, scientific literacy levels, cultural backgrounds, and professional fields'. Despite these odds, Professor Diaz was determined 'to teach all students Anatomy more effectively, in less time, and often with limited resources'.

Her teaching principles include:
- 'use of human cadaveric tissues'
- engagement theory, where students can participate 'in meaningful learning activities through interaction with others and worthwhile tasks'
- 'inclusiveness'; involving students across the healthcare profession spectrum
- teaching 'the learning skills that will serve them throughout their student and professional lives'
- adopting 'deep learning through understanding and the ability to place information into a broad, big picture which also makes it relevant to the students' realities'.

To achieve these ends, she introduced a range of innovative approaches that 'complement the use of prosected tissues', and are hands-on and without the use of lectures. The focal point is the laboratory, where 'team activities encourage

Multi-sensory learning by all students'. Being sensitive to individual learning styles, her methods involve whiteboarding and drawing, which 'is most appealing to visual learners', allowing students to summarise and synthesise concepts and facts and 'drawing anatomical structures'; use of Play-Doh, 'appealing to tactile learners', whereby students 'build anatomical structures using Play-Doh; [and participate in] movement, singing, dancing', where 'many students learn by doing … performing body movements with weights, a hula hoop; and surface Anatomy/ body painting'. Students 'consolidate what they learn with prosections … by looking at the surface anatomy relevant to the area on themselves, each other, or even family and friends'. Further, she notes that '[b]ody painting has become the most popular technique, as it is a very engaging way for students to learn Anatomy'. A crowning event at the end of the year is the 'anatomy Cup', 'as a friendly, fun, and stimulating inter-health discipline competition that give students a chance to showcase all these new approaches for learning Anatomy'.

What is perhaps most remarkable and gratifying is that students 'are achieving a >80% increase in the pass rate since 2005 and that the fail rate has dropped by 30%'.

Moreover, Professor Diaz's results for her 176 first-year health science students were better compared with the 155 medical students 'who do a separate more didactic Anatomy course'. A study on perception of the course found that her health sciences students 'were significantly more likely, than the medical students, to enjoy the subject, have higher-quality learning experiences, have a higher level of interest in the course, believe the teachings to be more relevant to their later years and professional career, and have a higher level of interaction with both their peers and teachers'. She consistently receives 4.1–4.6 on a 5-point rating scale regarding student interest, motivation and learning experience. Comments from her students are equally positive: 'Claudia is an inspirational teacher, her enthusiasm and love of anatomy is infectious, and the variety of techniques are fantastic learning aids.' She clearly demonstrates that interprofessional learning works. Besides, the learning experience can also be stimulating and enjoyable.

Learning that lasts: the 'law of cumulative ignorance'

By integrating a variety of teaching methods that are sensitive to the learning styles of the students, the teacher also ensures that the students are able to conceptualise, recall and apply the knowledge and skills they are gaining. And, while much has been written about the importance of aligning competencies with learning outcomes along with learning activities and assessments,[168] there are many stories in education at all levels where a mismatch has occurred between what students thought they were supposed to know and what they were actually tested on. In the most serious cases of what some have called 'educational malpractice' (e.g. failing final year examinations), students and parents have even taken schools and postgraduate institutions to court using the syllabi (learning outcomes) as a legal contract between the institution and the learner. In some fields, aviation for example, such misalignment could have disastrous consequences. We can only speculate the extent to which this misalignment could contribute to compromising safety in medical education (e.g. surgery).

However, less has been said about ensuring that the knowledge dimension of learning requires ongoing reinforcement to avoid what psychologists call 'extinction'. The 'law of cumulative ignorance' tries to explain what can happen to learners if they are allowed (or allow themselves) to forget, as shown in Figure 5.4, taking anatomy as an example. In a typical 5-year undergraduate programme, Figure 5.4 indicates the student did very well at the end of the first year, achieving 90% of the learning outcomes set for the year on the final examination. The student proceeds to Year 2 theoretically carrying at least 10% ignorance about anatomy – probably more, given summer holidays and other distractions. In Year 2 the student may now only achieve 80% on the final and the scenario continues. By the final year the student may actually fail anatomy as he or she has acquired about 60% 'ignorance'. While the 'law' is of course not really verifiable, as there are too many factors involved in the learning process, it does, however, make a point and it may ring true for those who recall being allowed to advance to higher levels in mathematics, physics or music although they were barely passing in their existing year.

From an educational perspective there may be benefits to consider wider use of pre and post testing each year, to determine what they already know at the beginning of a course (i.e. readiness to learn) and how well they have progressed during the year. The variance could also pinpoint specific areas of difficulty at individual and cohort levels that may need to be dealt with at the beginning of the following year.

The concept recalls the work of Vygotsky, Bruner and Piaget[135] and reinforces the importance of identifying top-level competencies (knowledge, skills, professional values and attitudes) that are deemed fundamental to meeting population or patient healthcare needs. Distinguishing between what is important may be facilitated by asking what 'must' be learned rather than what 'should' and 'could' be learned', if enough time and other resources were available.

It also suggests that the curriculum planners need to ensure that the curriculum structure allows for learning to proceed incrementally, systematically and repeatedly from the simpler levels to the more complex later, that is, adopting a spiral curriculum framework.

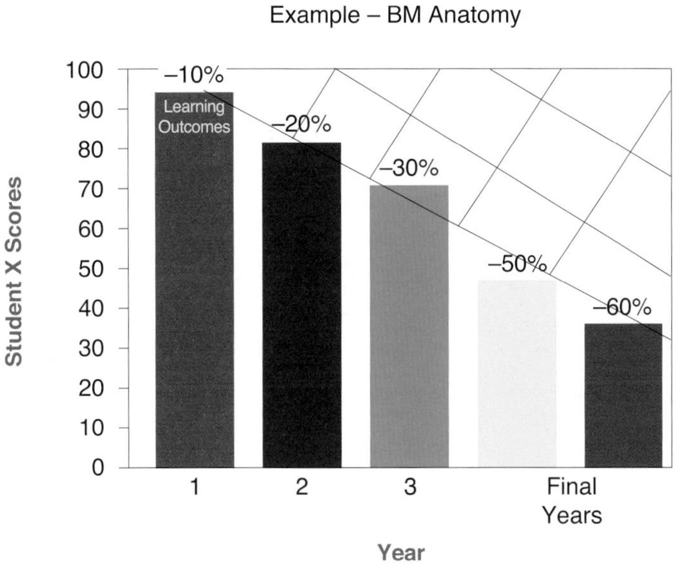

Example – BM Anatomy

FIGURE 5.4 Learning that lasts: 'the law of cumulative ignorance'

As Figure 5.5 shows, in the future more consideration may also be given to shifting from compartmentalised subject area medical education curriculum – with its continuing reliance on lectures and 'small' group discussions that often become mini-lectures – to integrated issue-centred learning and educating the whole person.

Changing the traditional 'teaching' formats could be facilitated by the shift toward competency-based approaches that allow 'for a highly individualised learning process rather than the traditional, one-size-fits-all curriculum. Ideally, students would have an opportunity to explore a range of choices in learning'.[56] As discussed in Chapter 3, competencies to be developed will need to be organised around twenty-first-century skills. In healthcare, these skills, which are in line with patient and healthcare system needs, will embrace both clinical and non-clinical competencies, especially 'higher order thinking skills, including critical thinking and problem-solving, research, collaboration and communication'.[143]

Further, these competencies will need to be shaped 'by adaptation ... to specific contexts drawing on the power of global flows of information and knowledge', to align 'national efforts through joint planning especially in the education and health sectors, engage all stakeholders in the reform process, extend academic learning sites into communities, develop global collaborative networks for mutual strengthening, and lead in promotion of the culture of critical inquiry and public reasoning'.[56]

Professor Dominic Shellard, vice-chancellor of De Montfort University in the United Kingdom, while commenting on higher education, may also have captured

Example

**Comparing Healthcare Practices in
the Developed and Developing World**

**1 Types of Health Problems
2 Current Treatments
3 Future Outlook...**

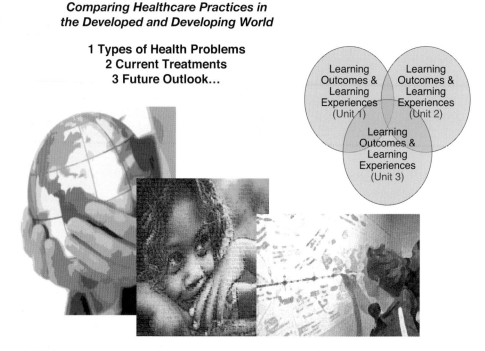

FIGURE 5.5 Learning inter/trans-professionally through theme and project-based approaches

the mindshift or 'spirit' that is necessary to restructure healthcare education and training, in order to meet patient needs in the early years of this century:

> In the next decade what matters is not the university motto, shield or history, but the thinking, attitude and creativity. We need the confidence to move beyond our comfort zone into new arenas, new areas of collaboration, new ways of working and thinking. To do so may threaten the old certainties about our identity, but it could also herald a renaissance for the perception of the academy in society.[169]

Medical education and the management of change

Improving postgraduate education: lessons from a national study

An example of the steep climb facing those who are keen to get on with improving medical education is well documented in a recent report of a national postgraduate medical specialist education reform in Denmark,[170] where changes in content and format of specialist education were introduced consistent with outcomes-based education. The comprehensive study involving approximately 3000 doctors and with excellent survey response rates (75%) after 3.5 years 'found limited impact on clinical training practice and learning environment'. The probability of implementing change was greater in the laboratory specialties compared with cognitive task (e.g. internal medicine, paediatrics, psychiatry) or technical task-oriented specialties (e.g. surgical, anaesthesiology, gynaecology). While the number of respondents who participated in courses on teaching and learning increased, attendees were usually junior doctors. Recommendations included focusing 'on changing the pedagogical competence of the doctors participating in daily clinical training'. The researchers also confirmed the importance of Professor David Wooton's argument in *Bad Medicine: doctors doing harm since Hippocrates* that implementing change in healthcare requires 'strategies for changing educational culture'.[171]

National Health Service cultures and organisational performance: research findings

Although the role of culture in organisations is contentious, Lee Bolman and Terrence Deal, both experts in leadership and organisational development, conclude that 'every organisation develops distinctive beliefs and patterns over time'.[172] For some, culture is simply 'the way we do things around here', while for others (e.g. Edgar Schein, a former professor at the MIT Sloan School of Management), culture goes beyond surface-level values and refers to 'the deeper level of *basic assumptions* and *beliefs* that are shared by members of an organisation, that operate unconsciously'.[173]

These beliefs are very much in evidence throughout the recent report *Changing Management Cultures and Organisational Performance in the NHS* (OC2).[174] The thrust of the study was 'to understand the nature of changing management cultures in the NHS and explore their relationships with changing organisational performance'. In doing so, Professor Russell Mannion *et al.* differentiate inter alia between four main cultural orientations that operate within NHS hospitals: (1) *Clan Culture* – 'cohesive, participative leader as mentor bonded by loyalty, tradition, emphasis on morale'; (2) *Developmental Culture* – 'creative, adaptive leader as risk-taker, innovator bonded by entrepreneurship emphasis on innovation'; (3) *Hierarchical Culture* – 'ordered, uniform leader as administrator bonded by rules, policies emphasis on predictability'; and (4) *Rational Culture* – 'competitive, acquisitive leader as goal-oriented bonded by competition emphasis on winning'. Whereas the Clan and Developmental cultures 'focus on flexibility, individuality and spontaneity', the Hierarchical and Rational cultures value 'control, order and stability'.

Their typology has direct implications for medical education that supports physicians working in these hospital environments whose work largely assumes that educational changes are optimised in Developmental cultures. Individuals who pursue values of the former culture tend to subscribe particularly to innovative approaches to learning and often advocate curriculum and delivery methods that are multidisciplinary and enquiry-based and that take advantage of informed research in the behavioural, psychological and neurosciences.[175]

A key finding of the report is that within the hospitals 'individual perceptions of culture have seen a marked shift across the time periods away from Clan orientations and towards (especially) Hierarchical and (to a lesser extent) Rational orientations'. However, this swing is not indicated at Practice level, where, perhaps unsurprisingly, with its emphasis on loyalty and tradition, 'the overwhelming dominance of Clan orientation shows no sign of diminution'. It is also noteworthy that 'in none of these professional groups was there evidence of a culture opposed to the dominant culture'. The managerial culture sees improvements occurring from a hierarchical or top-down approach, whereas practitioners, arguably, appear to have closed ranks and are responding by maintaining the status quo. None of the parties appear to have taken on a dominant Developmental mantle, which, arguably, is a prerequisite for change and innovation in healthcare education.

The preceding analyses point to at least two main hurdles that medical educators may need to consider in terms of advancing curriculum reforms at both undergraduate and postgraduate levels in developed countries. The first challenge is how major change will be possible when the tendency across medical units is toward maintaining 'tradition' within a dominant 'hierarchical' culture. The second major issue, as already discussed, is related to contemporary incoming medical student profiles, where preferences across the medical specialties indicate work expectations and behavioural norms that may be at odds with a world where openness, intuition, feelings, adaptability and informal relationships are increasingly required, rather supplanting inflexibility and depersonalisation.

The adaptive-generative development model to guide change and innovation[133]

While there are differences between the two, the implementation of change and innovation in research-led universities and in medical education seems to have much in common. In the last few years both have been tasked with focusing on the needs of the end user, student and patient, respectively; both have been under pressure to do more with less and both have to work things out in an uncertain and unpredictable world.

Enacting significant reform in either system is problematic, as there are increasingly competing priorities draining the energies of staff and limited coffers for organisations. Several years ago I wanted to address these issues, as there did not seem to be any helpful models to guide change efforts in academia. Most existing change models were too formulaic, corporate-directed, based on technical-rational problem-solving and without really capturing the essence of what it is like to lead and support change in complex social environments. In addition, most seemed incongruous in the light of a world where 'the issues we face … more often contain messes, divergent problems and conflicts of values which require systematic and creative ways of thinking and acting', and 'where creative, intuitive and critical processes are needed in order to develop new understandings'.[176]

One result of this research led to identifying factors (*see* Table 6.1) that, according to the literature, facilitate change and innovation in environments characterised by 'problematic goals, unclear technology and fluid participation'.[177]

The second outcome of this research was to formulate a framework for guiding change initiatives that incorporated these factors and that could be considered a useful aide-memoire, helping decision-makers to identify actual concerns or issues and to engage those affected by the change.

Fundamental to the design of such a framework was constructivist philosophy, which, in contrast to traditional logical scientific paradigms, and as far as human

TABLE 6.1 Summary of factors facilitating change and innovation[133]

Change dimension	Summative enabling factors
Development focus	Process (versus product)
Organisational culture	Balancing developmental-managerial norms and conservative-radical tendencies
Approach to change	Problem-solving
Role of change agent(s)	Process helper
Fundamental principles	Experiential/praxis Collegial/collaborative Credibility/meaningfulness Verification/multiple contexts Change as learning: adaptation and generative
Considerations for education	Systems approach to curriculum planning New technologies/critical reflection Cognitive models (versus behaviourist) Constructivism – personal meaning-making

learning is concerned, 'involves the construction of meanings in a continuous and active way'[178] and was a framework for change entitled the adaptive-generative development model of change (*see* Figure 6.1).[133] The philosophy is also informed by three primary propositions that originate in situated learning theory: (1) that learning is a function of the context in which it occurs, (2) that 'our personal world is constructed in our minds, and that these personal constructions define our personal realties' and (3) that the main stimulus for change is cognitive conflict or puzzlement.[179] Moreover, an important consideration of constructivism is that 'knowledge develops through social negotiation and through the evaluation of the viability of individual understandings'.[180]

Considered collectively, it seemed reasonable and appropriate to apply these premises to understanding the process of change, which is essentially a form of learning for the individuals involved and the organisation. The adaptive-generative development model, therefore, focuses attention on the duality of change: the need to adapt to existing conditions and the need to respond creatively to problems or issues. The underpinning philosophy that coheres the model is that change results from the shared construction of meaning made possible by a 'truly interactive, inclusive team'.[181]

Figure 6.1 advances that any anticipated transformative change must be solidly rooted in extensive *Needs Analysis* and *Research and Development*, one approach of which is seen through Bolman and Deal's multiframe lenses,[172] through which people see the world and make sense of it. According to the authors, the four main lenses or frames through which they try to interpret human interaction or phenomena include the structural frame (focusing on task, facts, and logic); the human resource frame (placing people first); the political frame (understanding the reality of the politics in the organisation); and, finally, the symbolic frame (drawing on social and cultural anthropology – based on ceremonies, rituals, rules, myths, policies, stories, heroes and managerial authority, and so forth). Multidimensional approaches are particularly important at a time when resources are tight and demand for new or better services are high and when 'restructuring' may push systems toward concentrating 'on competitive strengths and market niches, to eliminate weaknesses, to increase productivity and to enhance the strategic capacity … while devolving much autonomy to operating units'.[181]

Strategy Formation and Development requires 'thinking together' through the process of social negotiation and 'is likely to involve listening to voices that have not traditionally been at the centre of the decision process rather than favouring conventional [and dominant] views'.[181]

Resource Support necessitates the application of a multiframe strategy, for 'unless each issue is matched with an appropriate response, the intended changes will fail – or backfire'.[172] It also requires the building of a permanent resource capacity as '[g]etting a place on the real budget, or changing the way the real budget is allocated, represents real systemic change, and it is one of the greatest challenges to any change agent'.[182] Professor Andy Hargreaves, lead editor of the *Second International Handbook of Educational Change*,[183] suggested a number of approaches for gaining project funding and, although made several years ago, his advice may still ring true, especially in these times of financial constraints:

> Act politically to secure support and resources for the good of your students and, indeed, all students. … Use influence, persuasion, diplomacy, charm, self-mockery. Trade favours, influence power brokers, build coalitions, lobby for support, plant seeds of proposal before presenting them in detail, and find out how what you want meets the interests of others.[184]

Implementation and Dissemination usually follows the pattern 'packaging, diffusion, adoption and summative evaluation'.[185] As Fullan and Miles conclude, reform must focus on the development and interrelationships of all the main components of the system simultaneously, and not just on structure, policy and regulations but on deeper issues of the culture of the system.[186]

Evaluation of the effectiveness and efficiency of the change efforts lead back to the strategy formation and implementation processes and could also benefit from Bolman and Deal's four-dimensional processes[172] and how changes in one frame have impacted on the others.

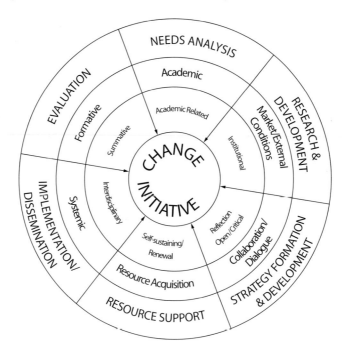

FIGURE 6.1 The adaptive-generative development model to guide change and innovation[133]

Enacting change: 'think globally, act locally'[56]

Traditionally, major educational reforms have been structural in content – often effected top-down. However, unfortunately, 'what emerges from evaluations of large-scale structural reforms is how little they impact below surface manifestations'.[187] One observation on change management comes from James Duderstadt,[188] former president of the University of Michigan, who points out that '[c]hange does not happen because of presidential proclamations or committee reports, but instead it occurs at the grassroots level of faculty, students and staff. Rarely is a major change motivated by excitement, opportunity, and hope; it more frequently is in response to some perceived crisis.'

While change intents are generally well founded, it is arguably a combination of strategic goals or systems thinking (linking global, national and local goals) and an awareness of change and educational development processes that may facilitate planning of educational interventions. Rather than following the adage 'form follows function', we often begin with structural considerations, when perhaps initially we should be paying considerably more attention to examining social, economic and cultural differences of our local surroundings, understanding and debating the nature of the aims, and gaining commitment by building collaborative relationships among those who will be affected by the change, many of whom may never have had the opportunity to work together or to challenge the thinking of centralised planning. This refocusing has been found to be particularly useful in the design of 'temporary educational systems'[175] that range from testing a new idea in a course to exploring new ways to plan, conduct and evaluate new programmes. The reforms being called for by national and international committees will certainly range across the five categories as shown in Figure 6.2, although the majority will most likely proceed through smaller curriculum change initiatives first, that is, at levels A or B.

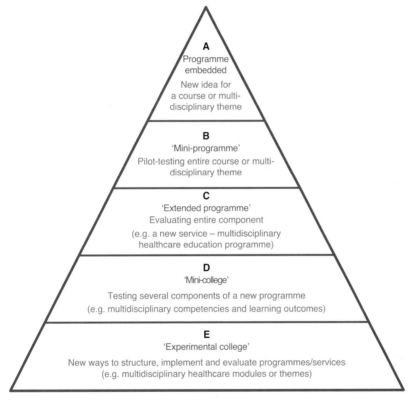

A
Programme embedded
New idea for a course or multi-disciplinary theme

B
'Mini-programme'
Pilot-testing entire course or multi-disciplinary theme

C
'Extended programme'
Evaluating entire component
(e.g. a new service – multidisciplinary healthcare education programme)

D
'Mini-college'
Testing several components of a new programme
(e.g. multidisciplinary competencies and learning outcomes)

E
'Experimental college'
New ways to structure, implement and evaluate programmes/services
(e.g. multidisciplinary healthcare modules or themes)

FIGURE 6.2 The temporary educational systems pyramid: guiding educational development projects[175]

Building an action culture

Figure 6.3 proposes a matrix for enacting academic change through developing an action culture. The framework, which has been previously applied in higher education,[166] juxtaposes two dimensions of change, articulated in the seminal literature on change management. On the horizontal axis are four principal change strategies,[189] while the vertical axis identifies three main types of educational development[190] activity. The matrix suggests that the first point of intersection should focus on building interpersonal trust (e.g. through interactional and collaborative leadership, open discussion, and social interaction at the level of the social or work group). The essential aim is to find consensus and agree the proposed change. Here it is important to recall that emotions often override reason and that personal gains and self-image play an important part in finding common ground. No one likes to be told it was all a mistake. History has shown that lasting change begins with a series of small steps that become increasingly larger as success is experienced. Another stage is to analyse the local environment – current and expected – in relation to the larger picture and to discuss the culture needed to bring about the changes and to match staff attributes and role expectations to the anticipated organisational culture, possibly applying temporary educational systems development phases,[175] including resourcing, implementing and evaluating the change.

The framework also advises that ideally the focus needs to be on curriculum issues and patient care, not politics or holding on to twentieth-century thinking. A good example lies with the issues identified by the international *Lancet*-commissioned study. There may be conservative or opposing forces but, while these need to be confronted, in the final analysis it is the patient in developed and developing countries who must take precedence over historical tradition or dated views.

For example, David Wooton, professor of history at the United Kingdom's University of York, concludes that '[h]ad microscopic research been actively pursued after the 1690s, traditional medical knowledge, and traditional medical

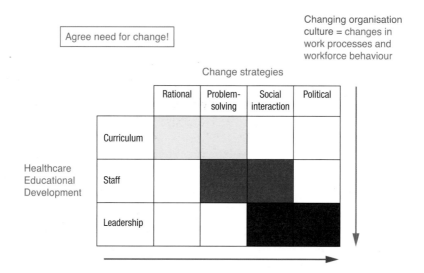

FIGURE 6.3 A matrix for enacting change: developing an action culture[117]

therapies, would have been under threat. Medicine had integrated the discoveries of the dissectionists and vivisectionists into medical education but the doctors refused to admit the relevance of the discoveries of the microscopists.' He argues, '[b]y turning their back on the microscope, they made it possible for traditional medicine to survive for a century and a half longer than it would have done had Leeuwenhoeck's discoveries been taken seriously.' He notes further that '[t]he opponents of the microscope did their job so successfully that even now the place of microscopy in the history of medicine goes largely unrecognised'.[171] Moreover, there is no doubt that one of the main reasons for the delays experienced in Britain in the late nineteenth century in regulating the medical profession – even though the Medical Act was passed in 1858 by the GMC – was the strife between the Royal colleges for most of the 30 years or so post 1858.

Interactional leadership: valuing emotions and social interaction

> Change is fundamentally about feelings; companies that want their workers to contribute with their heads and their hearts have to accept that emotions are central to the new management style … the most successful change programs reveal that large organizations connect with their people most directly through values – and that values, ultimately are about beliefs and feelings.[191]

Most likely identifying strongly with the latter observation, Knight and Trowler[192] proposed an approach to leadership that complements the academic change framework (*see* Figure 6.3), and one that differs from most others, as it places a high value on understanding the 'real issues' and 'feelings' of those who may be affected by the change. This type of leadership is based on social practice theory, which recognises that 'the most important aspect of change processes involves social interaction at the level of the workgroup'. The approach calls for a commitment to developing relationships built on trust and negotiation in order to develop 'understanding of the shape of departmental goals'.

The interactional leadership framework (*see* Figure 6.4), a key component of a more comprehensive adaptive-generative development model for change,[133] outlined earlier, and also applied previously in higher education in a cross-university study seeking to determine the extent to which educators rely on evidence practice to guide their decision-making,[166] may be useful to consider for progressing medical education initiatives. The model identifies three main stages: (1) inputs, (2) process and (3) outputs. Also, the model suggests adherence to social constructivist principles when leaders and teams embark on change.

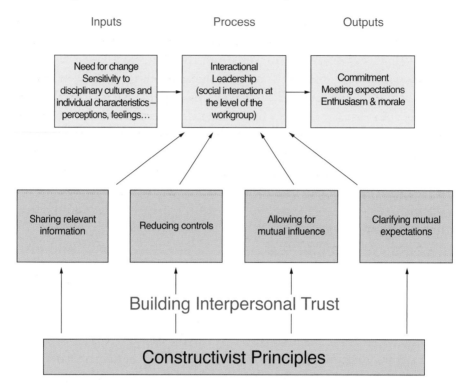

FIGURE 6.4 Interactional leadership framework: building interpersonal trust[166]

Applying the framework would involve consideration of not only the proposed change but also aspects related to understanding the target group's feelings and emotions regarding the change: dominant cultural orientations, staff morale and other sources to raise self-awareness. Anticipated outputs could include such measures as the change process itself, building trust, and clarifying priorities. Discussions with individual staff members or department teams would be underpinned by constructivist principles that value divergent views, evidence-based and anecdotal information, conceptual interlinking and social negotiation and collaboration.

Implications of applying the leadership framework in healthcare

In some areas this approach to change management in healthcare education could demand rethinking of staff appointment practices. One example is that the selection of department heads or coordinators would need to be carefully thought out, appointing candidates who have a strong track record in medical education, as well as ensuring that the successful candidate has at least the potential of realising the support of clinicians, other colleagues and learners. '[P]aying more attention to the social aspects of potential candidates' qualifications and experience' may increase the likelihood of satisfying this dimension.[193]

The importance of social aspects in medical education was confirmed in a qualitative study at Radboud University Nijmegen Medical Centre in the Netherlands, involving postgraduate nursing home physicians (N = 56) and supervisors (N = 62).[194] The researchers wanted 'to gain insights into the factors that influence the process of learning' and concluded that in four major domains (work environment, educational factors, student and supervisor characteristics) social integration was deemed to be most significant. Social integration was 'defined as a sense of belonging in the workplace or as a good atmosphere in which students felt integrated'. Two main factors impeded workplace learning: high workload and an unstable organisation, 'where the management structure is not clear to the student due to, for example, management problems or the merger of several departments'. Also, incumbents would need to demonstrate that they have the willingness to create opportunities for frequent interaction among clinicians, learners, and educators, tolerance of differences, generational and workload equity and consensus decision-making.[194] Finally, there is a case to be made for departmental or unit leaders to lead by example; one way could be to learn more about how change and reform take place at departmental or sub-departmental levels.[185]

Toward professional standards in healthcare education

A case in point relates to an initiative by the UK Academy of Medical Educators (AoME). Based on the rationale that '[d]eveloping a career in medical education is difficult', largely because of pressures from competing demands (service, research, regulators), a decision was taken to define knowledge, skill and values for medical educators that cut 'across national boundaries and disciplines'. 'What sets *Professional Standards*[195] apart,' say Professor John Bligh, dean of medical education as well as former president of the AoME, and Julie Brice, academic support manager, both at Cardiff University, is that the standards 'are applicable to all medical educators [including dentistry and veterinary sciences], whatever their background and area of expertise'.[196] The authors further suggest that the standards 'can be used by medical educators to monitor and plan their own development and by employers and others to assess individuals' performance'. Medical education is increasingly considered to be 'a clinical discipline in its own right with all the hallmarks of a clear area of professional practice', attracting clinicians who seek opportunities in medical education and leadership alongside their clinical roles.

'Choosing' to lead
· ·

The transition from practitioner to aspiring leader is not an easy one. However, as Ruth Collins-Nakai, cardiologist and chair at the Canadian Medical Foundation, points out, 'medicine focuses on decision-making at the individual physician-patient level'. 'Leadership', on the other hand, she reflects, 'necessarily involves stepping away from the individual-physician-patient relationship and examining problems at a systems level, requiring the ability to view issues broadly and systematically.'[197]

An advocate of 'learning by doing', Dr Collins-Nakai also notes that 'leaders of our current and future health care environment need not be high charisma individuals who create followers through personal magnetism. They can be people who have developed the skills of thinking and acting "outside the box," who can confront and challenge old patterns, and spearhead new ones, at any level.'

Dr Collins-Nakai cites Wiley Souba, dean of Dartmouth Medical School, whose fundamentals of 'physician leadership' include 'an inward journey of self-discovery and self development … clarity around a set of core values that guide the organization as it pursues its goals' and 'building a culture of excellence and accountability throughout the entire organization', while recognising that *'Leadership and learning are inextricably linked'*.[133,198] Dr Souba's focus on the importance of the 'inner self' as a basis for value formation in personal relationships and working life recalls the wise words on leadership of Lao Tzu, philosopher and founder of Taoism in the fifth century BCE:

> *To lead people, walk beside them …*
> *As for the best leaders, the people do not notice their existence.*
> *The next best, the people honor and praise.*
> *The next, the people fear; and the next, the people hate …*
> *When the best leader's work is done the people say,*
> *"We did it ourselves!"*[199]

> —Lao Tzu

The physician– patient contract

Changing physician–patient relationships

External factors will continue to impact on the shape of medicine in the coming decades, requiring careful monitoring and consideration. These developments may need to be given greater attention in undergraduate and postgraduate programmes – possibly within the 'hidden curriculum'. One of these is the 'physician–patient' contract. Jacalyn Duffin, a Canadian practising haematologist, educator and author, reminds us that historically '[a] contract has always existed between physician and patient, although usually it was not recorded in writing'.[200] Failure to meet expectations has ranged from the severe to 'fines, revocation of the licence to practice, and jail'. However, the patient–doctor relationship is changing to a large extent because of the public's awareness that there are limitations of medical knowledge and conflicting treatments.

Public perceptions of physicians

While the medical profession generally still enjoys high regard by the public in the United Kingdom, as far back as 1998, Sir Donald Irvine, then president of the GMC, noted three main concerns: (1) poor communication with patients and colleagues, (2) public perceptions of paternalism and (3) 'a suspicion, fuelled by some very public failures'.[99] It is noteworthy that these remain issues today as '[in] 2010 the top three types of concerns were about clinical investigations or treatment; respect for patients; and communication with patients'.[108] In the latest GMC surveys, there were also 'more complaints about male doctors, older doctors and GPs'.[108] While there are no simple answers, the problems are systemic and can likely be traced back, as discussed earlier, to the education and training of physicians.[56]

The United Kingdom is not alone in these, as Dr Duffin points out.[200] On both sides of the Atlantic there is growing public scepticism of 'class distinctions, authority and anything scientific' and '[w]hile society has come to expect miracle cures from medicine', she asserts, 'its expectations have declined to "low"'. Reasons for her observation are complex and include, as Sir Donald Irvine and most recently the GMC also mention, medical errors (e.g. tonsillectomy, surgery for visceroptosis, thalidomide); knowledge explosion and conflicting information; mistrust of 'medical heroes'; the fallibility of 'doctors'; and cure, which gradually became an important expectation, is now a right. 'As a result,' Duffin concludes, 'the contract between doctors and patients suffers from a double-bind. On the one hand is the cultural mistrust of medicine, science, and authority; on the other, a belief that every person has the right to a technological fix.' Perceptions of the medical profession or healthcare generally are certainly not helped by attention-grabbing headlines such as 'Nine-to-five GPs have lost trust of patients', 'Don't give out cancer drugs if it's just to extend life' or 'Patients go hungry in half of hospitals'.

Richard Smith, previous editor of the *BMJ*, presents several dimensions of how physicians have been viewed by patients and by themselves.[201] According to Dr Smith, patients have long regarded modern medicine as solving 'many of my problems – even social problems', whereas the doctor's belief, which Smith calls the 'bogus contract', recognises that modern medicine has limited powers, can be dangerous, can't solve all problems, especially social ones, and that 'the balance between doing good and harm is fine'.

The result of the latter perspectives, Smith feels, has led to 'disappointed, confused, misled, and sometimes angry patients; infantilisation of patients; unhappy, scared, defensive doctors; and people taking poor care of themselves, imagining that doctors can put them back together and with underutilization of self-management'.

Toward a new physician–patient contract

Responding to this quandary, Dr Smith proposes a new contract, one that encourages greater openness and public awareness and that acknowledges:
- death, sickness and pain are part of life
- medicine has limited powers, particularly to solve social problems
- people need to understand that medicine can be risky
- doctors don't know everything
- doctors too need decision-making and psychological support.

He further advocates that patients have to take more personal responsibility for their behaviour and should not leave problems to doctors. Supporting directions toward information age healthcare,[72] Smith also advises that the notion of 'we're in this together' needs to be strengthened – most likely in every consultation and certainly throughout medical education, including continuing professional development opportunities.

Basing his observations on medical case evidence, his overall message is that '[p]artnership with patients may lead to better outcomes, higher satisfaction, and lower costs'. Sir Donald Irvine posited over a decade ago that the patient as consumer has 'come centre stage' and 'for doctors used to being in the driving seat, that change can be difficult'.[99]

Promotion of Dr Smith's observations may be optimised in medical schools. There is no question that the content of medical education has changed considerably over the past few decades. However, while the medical content has changed, there may be two fundamental problems with how medical education is presently enacted. The first has philosophical underpinnings, while the second has more to do with clinical teaching practice and role modelling.

Most medical educators would likely agree that medicine is both an art and a science, and to become a competent and caring physician requires not only the acquisition of technical and adaptive skills but also a growing understanding of the human side of medicine; some would argue the most important factor in the healing process. However, the medical curriculum leans heavily toward the curative and biological model of disease, backed by tremendous progress in the science discoveries in the twentieth century and the past decade. These developments are captured in medical curricula to the point that most texts and syllabi focus on the science of medicine, and the message conveyed to students is, by and large, that what really counts or is valued most is mirrored in the examinations that decide who passes and who fails.

The term 'preventive' medicine, topics or interventions that may prevent illnesses or conditions from occurring in the first place, seldom appear in curriculum documentation and, arguably, less so in clinical lectures. An easy way to test this observation is to randomly select a curriculum document and search for the term 'preventive medicine' or its equivalent or to focus on important topics, such as cardiovascular subjects and to determine how much time is allocated to discussing factors that prevent heart attacks and strokes. So, while most medical schools espouse the need for the arts and humanities – for the development of 'humanitarian physicians', translating this thinking into practical reality is often fraught with great difficulty, as students find these 'soft' activities a distraction from the real business of medicine. Interpersonal and interprofessional activities are then frequently placed into the awkward position of justifying their existence in the curriculum. Consequences of the status quo may help to explain 'poor communication with patients' and 'paternalistic' attitudes identified in the GMC[108] and other studies.

This situation may be pervasive in other countries. 'Historically', say the three physicians and authors in a supplement to the *American Journal of Preventive Medicine*, 'the public health, population health, and prevention aspects of medical education were often omitted from physician training'.[202] However, they emphasise that 'efforts to develop health professionals who can improve health, and not just deliver health care, should be a continuing priority for academic medicine and public health communities'. Further, they assert '[t]here is an urgent need for physicians with a better appreciation for these issues to help address complex public health challenges that include rising chronic disease burdens, persistent health disparities, and healthcare financing that encourages treatment over prevention'. Writing in the same supplement, Dr John Prescott,[203] chief academic officer of the Association of American Medical Colleges, also argues for greater integration of public health and preventive principles and practices into medical education. In his view – and a major theme throughout this book – '[p]roducing better physicians for the future clearly requires a reconsideration of their education'. In the future, he notes, physicians must be 'skilled team players, who excel in systems-based practice, who provide patient-centred care, and who can work with and in their communities to improve health'.

It is possible that some of the answers for raising the commitment to support these directions may lie with finding out what motivates senior clinicians to teach medical students or trainees in the first place. Role modelling is likely the most powerful factor in shaping the beliefs and attitudes of future doctors. An Australian study[204] tried to investigate this question several years ago primarily with a view to improving 'the recruitment and retention of important clinical teachers'. Their study found that 'the main factors influencing motivation to teach medical students were intrinsic issues such as altruism, intellectual satisfaction, personal skills and truth seeking'. Reasons for not teaching 'included no strong involvement in course design, a heavy clinical load or feeling it was a waste of time'. According to the authors, an important point was that enhancing teaching engagement was 'within "the ownership" of universities' and that a key factor for improving recruitment, retention and motivation was involvement or inclusion of clinical teachers in course design, in particular if given '[o]pportunities to highlight special interests and to teach effectively'. The wish to be more involved in course design may be an opportunity to engage with small groups of students and to develop some understanding of student needs.

These discussions may also lead to identifying novel ways of strengthening communication and other interpersonal skills and possibly dealing openly with matters associated with the 'hidden' curriculum, such as the findings of reports or trends in medicine and changes in physician–patient relationships. The small group meetings, while likely difficult to arrange given 'the service burden amongst clinical teachers', appear to be essential in progressing the non-clinical education agenda, as the learners have the opportunity to engage with their clinical mentors in an informal and personal context, while the mentors get a first-hand opportunity to find out about student interests outside the clinical field and perceptions with respect to patients and, for example, working with colleagues in other specialty areas or other healthcare professions. Interestingly, the Australian study showed that 'contracts, money, a sense of duty and peer pressure play little part in motivating teachers', although there appears to be an 'important place of modest rewards such as Dean's teaching prizes'.

Overall, the inquiry concluded that recruitment and retention of clinical teachers is likely 'to have increased success if prospective teachers contribute to course development, sufficient time is allocated to teaching, memories of inspirational teachers are reawakened, the link between strong teaching and junior doctor outcomes is emphasised, and staff are reminded to advertise their specialty'.

Professional as 'authority': a patient's story

While there are many instances where the patient is the problem, there are also numerous examples when the fault lies with the doctor and where working as partners with patients – rather than as simply consumers of medicine – becomes essential. In a case reported in the *New York Times* a few years ago,[205] the patient's doctor 'correctly figured out what was wrong' with Ms Wong but refused to tell her. The test came back, and 'the doctor told her she had a virus. And to take the medicine for two weeks'. However, when she asked about the type of virus she had and how she got it, she was simply told to '[t]ake the medicine and come back in two weeks.' Two weeks later, she still felt ill and was told '[y]ou're fine, you're fine', and the doctor 'just patted her shoulder and sent her out', telling her to return in three months for another blood test. 'When she got her medical records, she learned that she had had hepatitis A, a viral liver infection.'

According to Gina Kolata, the well-known writer of the article, Ms Wong had come across

> a bane of the medical profession: the difficult doctor, who may be arrogant or rude, highhanded or dismissive. They drive away patients who need help, and some have been magnets for malpractice claims. And while such doctors have always been part of medicine, medical organizations say they fear that they are increasingly common – doctors, under pressure to see more patients, are spending less and less time with each one and are replacing long discussions

with laboratory tests and scans – and that most problem doctors apparently have no idea of their patients' opinions of them.

Kolata references Dr Beth A Lown, an assistant professor of medicine at Harvard Medical School and a past president of the American Academy of Physicians and Patients, who said: 'This goes to the heart of medicine – the skillful enactment of communication and a truly heartfelt understanding of the patient's circumstances. And it seems to have gotten lost as doctors get involved in medical systems that prioritize speed and technology. Increasingly, people are relying on tests instead of talking to patients.'

Both sides of the Atlantic have stories to tell. A very recent example of unprofessional behaviour in a UK hospital is disturbing. Two nurses – one an experienced paediatric nurse and mentor, the other, a nurse in training – had been looking after a month-old baby. Toward the beginning of the shift the doctor told the two nurses to remove the chairs they had placed for the distressed parents; at the end of the shift, the doctor – within hearing distance – advised the parents to disregard the nurses, as they 'did not know what they were talking about'.

This incident is troubling on several levels, as it shows a lack of professionalism and demeans the medical profession; it also demonstrates insensitivity to the feelings of the nurses, who had been trying (and had been working successfully) to save the life of a very young patient. In addition, it suggests to the community that collaboration among healthcare professionals is unimportant. Moreover, it calls attention to the fact that this type of authoritative and rude attitude is still common in modern healthcare practice, and that there needs to be a radical change in how healthcare professionals are selected, trained, socialised and recruited and how their performance is monitored. In addition, more attention needs to be paid to how staff and family members or carers at the receiving end of unprofessional behaviour should respond in situations like these.

Most patient–doctor agreements are implied, not express or stated 'in distinct and explicit language', 'except where a written informed consent is obtained'.[206] In the UK, as in other countries, guidance, such as the GMC's *Good Medical Practice*,[207] is provided on 'the principles and values on which good practice is founded'. Generally speaking, this type of guidance aims to inform medical professionalism but is not a regulated statutory code. Its other purpose is to let the public know what is expected of doctors. According to the GMC's *Good Medical Practice*, '[g]ood doctors make the care of their patients their first concern: they are competent, keep their knowledge and skills up to date, establish and maintain good relationships with patients and colleagues, are honest and trustworthy, and act with integrity'.[207]

Defining patient rights to good medical practice in the twenty-first century

Given recent cases of medical malpractice, of which the case relating to a month-old baby may be an example, professional regulatory bodies may need to reconsider how to strengthen patient rights. In California, for example, major health insurers initiated 'a new programme in which they divide US$30 million among 35,000 physicians depending on how their patients rate them'.[205]

Jo Charles[49] cites a report written 'by a number of medical leaders to envisage what it would be like to practise in a reformed NHS'.[208] The resultant design rules 'emphasise the importance of values; the nature of the relationship with patients and interaction with colleagues; the need for learning, measurement, and feedback in all systems; and that goals and targets for change need to talk about patients, and emphasise getting the basics right'.

She also references a report by the Picker Institute Europe[209] that could provide criteria or central metrics that patients, carers and healthcare providers may find useful in evaluating healthcare services.

- Fast access to reliable health service
- Effective treatment delivered by trusted professionals
- Participation in decisions and respect for preferences
- Clear, comprehensible information and support for self-care
- Attention to physical and environmental needs
- Emotional support, empathy and respect
- Involvement of and support for family and carers
- Continuity of care and smooth transitions.

Professional as 'partner': a junior doctor's story

In this story a junior doctor reflects on her shadowing experience. Having spent five minutes with a middle-aged man with a chronic disorder who had been in and out hospital for the better part of his life, the junior doctor imagines what it might feel like to be an inpatient 'with a full package of round-the-clock care'.[210]

> Lying alone in a dark stuffy side-room – abandoned by the powers that be, by the busy nursing staff desperate to avoid the foul-smelling wound, by the busy catering staff who can sail by without a minute's thought and by the busy doctors who think that they understand what is best. Can they even comprehend being in these shoes and surviving one day only to roll into one the next with more needles, more tests, more surgery, more pitying disdained faces and more suffering? I mean – how long does it take to smile, to ask me

how I feel, to spare a minute to explain or even give me a choice? I wish I was someplace else – anywhere but here, anywhere but this dark stuffy side-room, anywhere but alone.

For this trainee doctor, the patient–doctor contract needs no spelling out, as she seems to have an innate sense of what is expected of a good doctor. In her present world she expresses the hope that a 'good F1 [Foundation Year 1] doctor will spot these patients and give them enough so they are no longer that helpless depersonalised individuals on a hospital ward'. Moreover, she notes that this may mean 'staying five minutes longer after work and meeting your friends down the pub a bit later; perhaps it even means putting on a sympathetic face when all you want is to scream and get out of the building and be normal "Joe Bloggs" again because you're fed up with moaning patients'. She goes right to the central issue relating to the implicit physician–patient contract, when she notes: '[p]erhaps it means remembering why you wanted to be a doctor in the first place and actually doing that job justice'.

Along with patient-centredness and increasingly recognising the importance of the human side of patient care, other significant directions that are impacting on health professionals, as discussed at some length in this book, relate to the blurring of roles and the importance of teamwork as a basis for holistic support. The shift toward interdisciplinary healthcare teams supporting individual patients and social care agencies in communities will also require rethinking of the traditional physician–patient relationship. In future, the latter may depend much more on interdependent multi-care support teams functioning holistically at local levels and meeting personal needs that span health, social and possibly financial support roles.

In the United Kingdom, a recent report,[211] commissioned by the Royal College of GPs and the Health Foundation charity, if endorsed, provides specific markers for these types of shifts, which are essentially paradigmatic in scope.

The Commission recommends 'that "generalists" – usually GPs – need to look at the person as a whole as well as their family and home life rather than just particular diseases they may suffer from'. Further, as the population ages and more people live with long-term conditions, it recommends that 'doctors make themselves available around the clock, get to know patients over many years and help them with social problems as well as medical ones.'

While '[m]aking health needs assessments, addressing health inequalities and commissioning services accordingly are key components of this kind of approach', so, too, say the Commission members, 'is being known in the community (whether a physical community or a patient cohort), the obverse of the patient being known to the doctor'.[211] Children are said to have 'the least continuity of service ... partly because they are only ever seen as having short-term urgent needs, and their care is made worse because fewer than half of GPs have paediatric training'.

The Commission also calls for '[g]eneralists to make more and better use of new information and communication technologies to improve communication between them and their patients, and with other clinical professionals'.

Also, 'people with learning disabilities and elderly people living in care homes also receive an especially poor deal,' and the report recommends that all care homes should have 'dedicated GPs responsible for their residents .... Another factor blamed for doctors neglecting broader care for patients is the 'straightjacket' of targets and bonuses for treating and preventing particular diseases.[212]

Further, consistent with *The Lancet* Commission[56] and World Health Organization conclusions,[80]

> the report says more doctors will need to become generalists as the ageing population means that more patients suffer from long-term conditions and have more than one disease at any time. But many young doctors are 'lured' into specialisms that are seen as more prestigious, while advances in science and technology has meant that generalism 'has risk extinction in many hospitals'.

Without a doubt, the Commission advocates 'high-quality generalism', but it is noteworthy that it was not 'able to conclude that generalism, as practised currently in the UK [unlike in Canada, for example] delivers as much for patients as it could'.[211] A root cause, as argued throughout this book, and now confirmed as well by the Royal College of GPs, lies in the education and training of medical students and trainees.

> Medical training needs to become much more generalist in content, with more of it taking place in primary care settings. A placement in general practice should be compulsory during the two-year foundation programme for medical graduates.
>
> There should be an immediate extension of the length of specialist training for GPs from three to five. *This must include specific provision for training in disciplines particularly relevant in general practice, including paediatric care, learning disability, mental health, care of people with life-limiting conditions, and end-of-life care for patients and their families.* In the short term, general practices should ensure they are able to draw on the expertise of doctors with special interests in these groups. All medical undergraduates should have greater experience of these core disciplines and opportunities for shared training modules across health and social care should be pursued.[211] (italics added)

It seems remarkable how some articles written more than a decade ago can still feel fresh and vital today. This includes a paper written by Sir Donald Irvine,[99] which covered most issues of the day and most of the present day – rising costs of healthcare, ethics, consumerism, interprofessionalism, public perceptions and move to greater explicitness, among others – and seems as relevant today as it was then. The wheels of change in medical education really do move slowly!

For example, he observed that 'since most of us now practise in multi-disciplinary teams, the notion of multi-professional collective responsibility is beginning to take shape and be explored', involving 'general practice, or the clinical team, department or directorate in hospital'. He also stressed that '[i]t is the medical profession's responsibility to see that professional practice is at one with people's expectations and that self-regulation really is effective'. The latter expectation remains to be achieved in most countries surveyed by the Commonwealth Fund study[54] and confirmed in *The Lancet*-commissioned report.[56]

While most of the issues raised by Sir Donald Irvine reverberate presently with a few more being added, Dr Duffin advises that '[q]uestions are now being asked about physician incomes, patient entitlements, and the allocation of costly instruments and procedures.' Further, she suggests that '[e]conomists and policy makers point to the tremendous savings that could result from concentrating our efforts on the prevention of heart disease, stroke, and lung disease, rather than waiting to deal with the consequences'. There are also serious moral issues. For example, she cites those who question 'the global inequities of spending millions of dollars to prolong the lives of elderly, sedentary, and well-heeled North Americans while thousands of children die every year from malnutrition and simple infections'. She states that '[t]hose who control the purse strings recognise that the more doctors there are, the more they cost'. A future physician–patient contract needs to give substantially greater emphasis to the principles of prevention rather than solely the continuance of the medical model of disease, 'which must be reconciled with providing optimal care for the majority at minimum cost'.[200]

In an insightful article for the *New York Review of Books*, Dr Richard Horton, editor-in-chief of *The Lancet*,[213] references a book by Jerome Groopman, Dina and Raphael Recanati chair of medicine at Harvard Medical School. Dr Groopman writes for the *New Yorker* and in his book delivers a sharp and 'coherent critique of medicine's mistaken direction'.[214] According to Horton, Groopman claims, 'there is a common flaw that undermines much of contemporary medical education and training, as well as the partnership between patient and doctor and even the professional values of medicine. That flaw lies in the way doctors think. … Whereas once they would take part in challenging and detailed debates about the patients they met and examined on rounds, they now "too often failed to question cogently or listen carefully or observe keenly. … Something was profoundly wrong with the way they were learning to solve clinical puzzles and care for people."' Disapproving of 'medical scientism', Groopman is also wary of doctors' over-reliance on evidence-based medicine, suggesting that '[o]ften patients have conditions or combinations of conditions that do not easily match the supposed evidence'.

Further, Horton, in referencing Groopman, highlights that '[o]n average, about 15 percent of a doctor's diagnoses are inaccurate' and a doctor 'more often than not fails to investigate why these diagnoses are missed. Doctors are rarely taught to ask how an error could have taken place, let alone how it could be avoided in the future. Most are unaware of their mistakes' and are 'uncertain about their own uncertainties' with 'alarming research that shows the worse their performance, the more certain they seem to be that they are right!' In Horton's view, Groopman 'reserves some of his most bitter criticism for his colleagues within academic medicine', where '[t]hey have fostered a belief that anyone can take care of patients', and where '"arrogance" has created a culture at academic medical centres where research is applauded and teaching is taken for granted, where writing scientific papers (for journals like *The Lancet*) takes precedence over developing clinical skills'.[213]

Moreover, according to Horton, Groopman's most radical proposition – from the doctor's point of view, anyway – is that the physician should seek a new ally in helping to correct the cognitive errors and biases inherent in his makeup. This new ally is the patient. Patients can ask questions that pull doctors away from the traps they might otherwise fall into.'

Finally, and central to this chapter, Groopman raises the question, 'What makes a good doctor?' In the past, the doctor 'professed a commitment to levels of competence and integrity that he expected society to respect and trust. This commitment formed the basis for a social contract between the profession and the rest of the community. In return for the moral values, knowledge, and technical skills displayed by doctors, society bestowed on them the authority, autonomy, and privilege to regulate themselves.' However, Groopman asserts, '[t]his version of professionalism is now moribund'. In contrast to the past, today, 'in many Western countries women now outnumber men at medical schools. The public is also far more educated than it was a century ago. Patients have access to the same information as doctors. They may know more than most doctors about their own condition.' And, although taking final responsibility for patient care, 'doctors increasingly work in teams. Their responsibilities are shared with many other professionals – nurses, therapists, and pharmacists.' Fundamental to being a doctor, Groopman emphasises, are the following: '[c]ompetence, knowledge, judgment, commitment, vocation, altruism, and a moral contract with society'.

A major distinction in the physician–patient relationship from previous generations is that '[t]he patient is a far more powerful force in a doctor's professional life today than in past generations. The patient expects to be more the equal partner of the doctor. Medicine's goal is not only to cure or palliate disease. It is also to promote a person's well-being and dignity. Many patients want to be engaged participants in a doctor's thinking, not just its passive recipients. Whereas once doctors spoke of the doctor–patient relationship, they now increasingly talk of the patient–doctor interaction.'

In terms of what makes a good doctor, citing Groopman, Horton's summary is particularly relevant to the themes in this book:[213]

> Good doctoring is about listening and observing, establishing a trusting environment for the patient, displaying authentic empathy, and using one's skills and knowledge to deliver superb care. But a neglected aspect of this professionalism is getting doctors to think about their own thinking. Only by doing so are doctors likely to reduce the number of errors they make. What should they do?
>
> Encouraging patients to tell and retell their stories is essential. 'Patients' fears about what might be wrong or their anxieties about the future course of their illness should be drawn out into the open. Whatever the doctor's own attitudes about the patient, it is a critical element of any mutually respectful therapeutic partnership that the doctor acknowledges the patient's version of the truth of his or her story. This acknowledgment may mean repeating tests or reconsidering a long and strongly held diagnosis.

Moreover, Horton states that Dr Groopman[213] cautions doctors

> [i]n their encounters with patients, irrespective of the financial incentives to be more efficient and productive, doctors must try to remain systematic and thorough when they take a patient's history and conduct physical examinations. Shortcuts are dangerous. Thinking requires the investment of time. Groopman repeats the same lesson again and again: slow down. The more time a doctor takes, the fewer cognitive errors he will make. ... And once a decision is made, always retain an element of doubt. That sliver of uncertainty will leave the doctor not only better able to recognize failure early but also free to revise his opinion as new information comes to light.

A common theme that weaves through this chapter has to do with quality of service for patients, which in turn requires a 'professional' approach to healthcare. In the United Kingdom the Health Secretary, Andrew Lansley, recently announced 'a new system to assess success in the health service based on the quality of care patients receive – not merely the speed at which they are treated'.[215] With a view to improving standards, the government will be monitoring and publishing comprehensive data 'on hospital death rates, the individual performance of GPs and surgeons and patients' experiences under their care'. Success in the NHS will be defined by 60 benchmarks that include 'a commitment to preventing unnecessary early deaths, a pledge to enhance the quality of life of people with long-term conditions and a drive to ensure that people have a positive experience when using the health service'. The Health Secretary argues that '24,000 early deaths a year could be prevented from cancer and other long-term conditions'. In a move that sees hospital care increasingly shifting people with 'long-term conditions including asthma and diabetes' to community care, there will be fewer people treated in hospitals.

While the initiative may be well intentioned, it has the potential of repeating past centralised attempts to regulate professions by setting new targets, when arguably these should be self-regulated or set by those who are directly responsible for patient care and safety. The difficulty with the latter view is that many systemic issues remain – waiting times, treatment of the elderly, methicillin-resistant *Staphylococcus aureus*, postponement of surgery, poorly trained healthcare assistants, to name but a few. One may question why these issues have been allowed to fester for so long in some hospitals. A positive side to the initiative is that rather than setting 'arbitrary targets' for healthcare, the government will in future be relying more on comparative clinical data to determine whether rates in 'cancer, liver and heart disease are improving', and use this information to underpin changes. Another benefit is that more weight is being placed on the 'patient voice' – in particular, in terms of the quality of care received and the speed of care. There can be little doubt that those clinical contexts – hospital/community, urban/rural – that consistently perform well on the 60 benchmarks will be allowed greater powers of self-regulation than those contexts that do not. Also, treating chronic conditions at the community level should make patient care more personalised and more cost-effective. The 60-step plan also seems to resonate with the Royal College of GPs and the Health Foundation charity report calling for lengthier training periods for GPs, who will be at the forefront of patient care in the community, necessitating 'upskilling' in particular areas or conditions.[211]

Although we have come a long way from the loose and uncoordinated system of healthcare that flourished until the late nineteenth century, as these stories, studies and measures illustrate, difficult hurdles remain. The biggest challenge may be fostering professional values or dispositions that place the welfare and well-being of patients at the forefront of patient care. It may depend on the new generation of doctors and other healthcare professionals to try to solve many of these issues. With a revitalised 'patient–healthcare professional' relationship in mind, *The Lancet* commissioners advocate the development of 'a set of common attitudes, values and behaviours' to complement their learning of specialties of expertise with their roles as accountable change agents, competent managers of resources, and promoters of evidence-based policies' along with:

enlightened new professionalism that can lead to better services and consequent improvement in the health of patients and populations. In this way, professional education would become a crucial component in this shared effort to address the daunting health challenges of our times, and the world would move closer to a new era of passionate and participatory action to achieve the universal aspiration for equitable progress in health.[56]

Realising the aims of medicine in the twenty-first century

Patients in the twenty-first century

To counter some of the public scepticism and help take medicine into the twenty-first century, proposed changes in healthcare are under way in many countries, including Britain. According to Lord Crisp,[216] former chief executive of the NHS and Permanent Secretary of the Department of Health (2000–06) and a *Lancet* report commissioner,[56] '[t]he biggest need and the biggest cost is to provide continuing help for older people with long-term conditions to look after themselves, manage intermittent crises and maintain their health and independence'. As things stand, he advises, 'the NHS is still a service that is geared more towards one-off episodes of hospital treatment than to providing community support. Both are needed but the balance has to change.'

As part of a major health and social care reform, 'broadly welcomed by the UK Royal College of Physicians and the Royal College of Surgeons', around 140 GP-led clinical commissioning groups (CCGs), which would include representation not only from GPs but also from other health and social care professions, are proposed to replace primary care trusts to 'make the NHS sustainable for the future'.[217] According to Dr Tim Thursten, elected to a CCG, the CCG's main focus will be to 'make decisions about patient care and how the NHS can best meet the population's needs'. The CCGs will be responsible for commissioning and managing 'a wide range of local health services including those at the big hospitals as well as commissioning community and prescribing services'. Once implemented, the CCGs will have 'to make difficult choices about how severe a problem needs to be before free care is justifiable and what the NHS should no longer be doing at all'.

Proposed reforms in the UK and other nations[56,101,104] are indicative of the extent to which these countries recognise that medical care will need to be delivered fundamentally differently from what is occurring at present, resetting essentially the relationship between 'three major groups of protagonists – the medical profession, consumers, and the state', as Jane Lewis, professor of social policy at the London School of Economics,[218] outlined several years ago. In her view, the tension stems from opposing views of the aims of medical care in a modern society – ranging from the doctor's 'absolutist ethic of treatment' to the state's concern for utilitarianism, and the belief that 'the profession needs to work not only for the individual but also for the collective good'.

The establishment of national health systems (e.g. Germany, 1883; Britain, 1911 and 1948 [NHS]; Canada, 1984) were designed to do just that.[200] Unlike developing countries, most European nations now have government-supported healthcare systems. However, in the United States, as mentioned in Chapter 1, there are presently about 46 million people who are uninsured, a situation that President Obama is trying to resolve with the passage of the Patient Protection and Affordable Care Act on 23 March 2010.[217] While '[i]ncreasingly US doctors are committed to the concept of coverage for all its citizens', Jacalyn Duffin points out that 'some are concerned about what might be at stake for them personally. Others who oppose the changes worry about their incomes and their freedom as professionals should the president succeed with "Canadian-style," "government-run," single-payer health care.' She cites an American physician-Congressman who sees 'the proposals as having the potential to destroy jobs, explode the deficit, ration care, and take away "the freedom American families cherish."' This doctor was certainly not speaking on behalf of the 46 million who are uninsured in the United States or the families of those who lost their children 'in a 1990 measles epidemic in Texas' because none had been vaccinated and were 'black and Hispanic children living in poverty'.[220]

'The purpose of these health care systems,' according to Dr Duffin[200] – 'be they private or public – is threefold: first to remove the onus for payment from the sick or the poor; second, to ensure that health-care services are remunerated; and third to prevent disease.' While the first two goals are often met; the third is not. In her view the term '"[h]ealth-care system" is a euphemism for managing and paying the wages of disease'.

The premise behind the changes advocated in national and international reports seems to be that we need not only to do things better – that is, enact first-order or evolutionary change, as shown in Figure 8.1A – but also to do better things, by transforming what currently exists or through innovation or second-order change processes, as illustrated in Figure 8.1B.

The latter type of approach is more radical, as it usually tries to address urgent issues. Those involved in institutional and instructional change of this magnitude may initially experience decreasing productivity with lower staff morale, but, as evidenced in other large-scale projects, over time when the changes have been embedded both morale and productivity increase and frequently at a higher level than before the intervention, as depicted in Figure 8.1C.

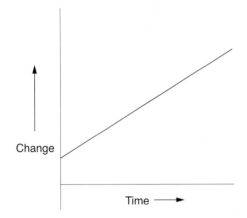

FIGURE 8.1A Evolutionary change

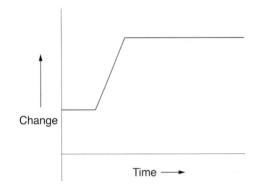

FIGURE 8.1B Transformational change

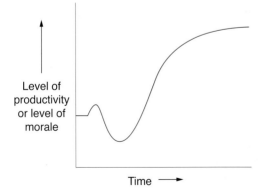

FIGURE 8.1C Successful innovation and the change curve

Role of medicine: cure illness, extend life or 'medicalise' society?

While calls for reform inspire many practical considerations, there remain even more philosophical and vexing questions about the central aim of medicine in this century – is it, as the late Roy Porter,[221] eminent British medical education historian, suggested, to cure or to prevent illness to keep people alive as long as possible? Or is it to fulfil whatever fantasies its clients may frame for their bodies? Are we falling prey, as Porter pondered over a decade ago, to 'an expanding medical establishment, faced with a healthier population of its own creation, is driven to medicating normal life events (such as the menopause), to converting risks into diseases, and to treating trivial complaints with fancy procedures?' Are '[d]octors and "consumers" alike ... becoming locked within a fantasy that unites the creation of anxiety with gung-ho "can-do, must-do" technological perfectibilism – everyone has something wrong with them, everyone can be cured?'

What Porter referred to is of course the 'medicalisation' of society – that is, 'the process of defining an increasing number of life's problems as medical problems'. In one of his presentations – as former editor of the *BMJ* – Richard Smith[201] gives several examples of medicalisation, noting in particular the increasing preference for caesarean births and, regarding death, 'with people wanting to die at home but mostly dying in hospital'. Some of the issues surrounding the medicalisation process include situations where people are treated 'when they are normal', the devaluing of 'non-medical interventions', people seeing themselves as 'victims' and perhaps failing 'to take action' themselves. Two key ways to counter medicalisation, according to Smith, are (1) to '[e]ncourage debate and understanding of medicalisation' and (2) to 'resist the constant growth in health budgets'.

Medicalisation is not confined to physical health. Phillip Collins, a writer for *The Times* and a senior visiting fellow in the Department of Government at the London School of Economics, in an informative article[222] traces the dreadful history of mental health – 'a litany of cruel failure' – in the United Kingdom and, in particular, raises the question 'how it can be that schizophrenics – invented by Swiss psychiatrist Eugen Bleuler in 1911 – are still treated in a way that would appal us if they had a visible, physical illness'. In the 1930s interventions included insulin injections, electroconvulsive therapy and lobotomies, involving 'smashing a sort of icepick through the top of each eye socket, severing the nerves that connect the frontal lobes to the part of the brain that controls emotional response'. In the intervening years drugs have been prescribed, '[f]irst sedatives such as barbituates, then palliatives such as lithium and valium'. However, Phillip Collins notes, '[e]ven when they calm everyday anger the drugs have no impact on the underlying condition. For lots of people, they are a slow lobotomy.'

Collins also laments the fact that while '[m]ental illness is more common and more costly than cancer', the illness 'attracts a fraction of the research, money or sympathy'. Further, he observes '[t]here is not a single physical condition in which recovery in the developed world trails the developing world, but it does in mental illness. It's an astonishing and shaming fact.' Referencing the controversial *Doctoring the Mind: is our current treatment of mental illness really any good*,[223] by the clinical psychologist Richard Bentall, the *Times* journalist highlights 'the success rate of drug-based psychiatry in treating serious psychoses and found it was not much better than the old astrologers and apothecaries'. An important part of the reason, as Dr Bentall explains, is because of the massive financial forces of the drug companies, whose influence on research, treatments and medical practitioners is pervasive. Dr Bentall notes that it is common among psychiatrists to medicate for life those who have been diagnosed with serious psychoses when more may not be better. Contributing to medicalisation of society in the United States is prescribing antipsychotic drugs for children who demonstrate 'disruptive' behaviour and for other emotional states such as grief or disappointment, which are frequently treated with serotonin-reuptake inhibitors.

Similar alarming trends and figures are appearing in Canada, where Rob Wipond reports 'nearly half of all seniors in long-term care in BC [British Columbia] are being given antipsychotics like Risperdal, Zyprexa and Seroquel. That's almost twice the average for the rest of Canada and amongst the highest rates found anywhere in the world.'[224]

An investigation by UK's Channel 4 *News* and reported by Kate Loveys, an education reporter for *The Daily Mail*, found that '[a] staggering 15,000 children under the age of 18 [compared with 7649 in 2001] were prescribed psychotic drugs last year by their GPs'.[225] Of these, most (11 451) were in the age group 13–18 years. Drugs, such as Risperdal and Seroquel are meant for serious mental conditions such as schizophrenia and bipolar disorders and psychosis, but experts feel that 'they are increasingly used to control children's behaviour, for example, to calm youngsters with attention deficit hyperactivity disorder or autism'. In the same article, Professor Peter Tyrer, an antipsychotic expert of Imperial College London, observes that the use of this medication is 'a slow fuse to disaster'. These figures follow other studies that revealed 'that 661,500 prescriptions for Ritalin or similar drugs for ADHD [attention deficit disorder] were issued to children last year' – amounting 'to more than 12,000 prescriptions per week and an increase of 70% in the past five years'.

While these drugs are prescribed, all too easily, it seems, with unknown long-term side effects and with 'pharmaceutical companies [blocking] all requests for data on trials involving children',[225] a question that needs to be asked is whether the prescriptions are doing any good and whether there are better alternatives. From this point of view, Dr Bentall's finding that 'schizophrenics in poor countries were doing a lot better than those in rich countries' should be of interest to parents and carers, as well as to government regulatory bodies such as the United Kingdom's Royal College of Psychiatrists. According to the writer, the difference may be attributed to how mental illness has been turned into a 'system', and that patient care may be 'better provided by former patients and … peers than by doctors and nurses'. The present approach places

> people into diagnostic groups according to the symptoms and then say that they are cured only when they disappear. If we define recovery as the capacity to live a meaningful life even as the symptoms persist (which is what, in effect, happens in countries with less expensive services) people tend to get better. Giving mental health patients a sense of control is a big factor.

Closely linked to Bentall's, Wipond's and Lovey's observations, and equally as disturbing, are the findings of a study in the United States, funded by the Congressional Office for Technology Assessment (now closed), of a group of five researchers, three of whom are physicians, about the dangers of conventional medicine.[226] In making their argument, the researchers point out that

> US health care spending reached $1.3 trillion in 2003 [*now over $2 trillion!*] representing 14% of the nation's gross national product. Considering this enormous expenditure, we should be preventing and reversing disease, and doing minimal harm. Careful and objective review, however, shows we are doing the opposite. Because of the extraordinarily, technologically driven context in which contemporary medicine examines the human condition, we are completely missing the larger picture.

Their fully referenced and meticulous report

> shows the number of people in the US having in-hospital, adverse reactions to prescribed drugs to be 2.2 million per year. The number of unnecessary antibiotics prescribed annually for viral infections is 20 million per year. The number of unnecessary medical and surgical procedures performed annually is 7.5 million per year. The number of people exposed to unnecessary hospitalisation annually is 8.9 million per year.

According to the researchers,

> [t]he most stunning statistic, however, is that the total number of deaths caused by conventional medicine is an astounding 783,936 per year … (By contrast, the number of deaths attributable to heart disease in 2001 was 699,697, while the number of deaths attributable to cancer was 553,251.5).

Further they argue, and as evidenced in Chapter 1, that medicine is not taking into consideration the following critically important aspects of a healthy human organism:

- stress and how it adversely affects the immune system and life processes
- insufficient exercise
- excessive caloric intake
- highly processed and denatured foods grown in denatured and chemically damaged soil
- exposure to tens of thousands of environmental toxins.

And, the authors maintain '[i]nstead of minimising these disease-causing factors, we cause more illness through medical technology, diagnostic testing, overuse of medical and surgical procedures, and overuse of pharmaceutical drugs. The huge disservice of this therapeutic strategy is the result of little effort or money being spent on preventing disease.'

Their overall conclusion is that '[a] definitive review of medical peer-reviewed journals and government health statistics shows that American medicine frequently causes more harm than good'.

Jerome Groopman, cited earlier, posits that one of the difficulties in realising the fundamental aims of medicine is the result of 'the errors and biases that most doctors unconsciously succumb to when thinking about what their findings mean for a patient's diagnosis and treatment.[214] In his review of Groopman's compelling book *How Doctors Think*, Richard Horton focuses on the cognitive errors that doctors make, including *attribution error* ('seeing the patient from only one – and often very negative – perspective, independent of what the clinical findings suggest'); *availability error* (making 'a decision based on an experience that is at the forefront of his mind but which bears little or no relation to the patient before him'); *search satisfying error* ('looking for an answer to the patient's problem as soon as he discovers a finding that satisfies him, albeit incorrectly'); *confirmation bias* ('when the doctor selects only some parts of the information available to him in order to confirm his initial judgment of what is wrong'); *diagnostic momentum* (when the doctor is unable to change his mind about a diagnosis, even though there might remain considerable uncertainty about the nature of a patient's condition'); and, finally, *commission bias* ('when the doctor prefers to do something rather than nothing, irrespective of clinical clues suggesting that he should sit on his hands').[213]

Unfortunately, so says Groopman,[214]

> [d]octors are not routinely taught these cognitive pitfalls. Nor are they trained to learn from their effects. Yet these errors and biases can prove fatal. Most doctors are unaware that their thinking is prone to predictable mistakes. Our

systems of medical practice neither seek to detect these mistakes nor feed their lessons back to doctors to prevent their recurrence.

Further, Horton points out Groopman's observation that '[d]espite his greater knowledge, the specialist is not immune from these missteps. Specialization can confer undue and sometimes dangerous confidence in those who possess such knowledge.'[213]

Mirroring the findings of the Congressional Office of Technologial Assessment study,[226] Groopman asserts that '[e]lectronic decision aids – devices that supposedly help doctors to arrive at the correct diagnosis – are unlikely to help, even though many extravagant claims are made for the impact of information technology on health'. Further, he 'believes such electronic fixes might actually encourage more mistakes. They are a distraction. They promote a reductive and unthinking kind of checklist behavior. And they divert the doctor away from what should be his primary focus: the patient's own story.'[214]

While effective communication is crucially important, Groopman's main argument is that

> [d]octors must also learn to think differently. A solid base of medical knowledge is not enough to be a good physician or surgeon. Research into cognitive errors in medicine reveals that most mistakes are not technical. They stem from mistakes in thinking. Intuition, a clinical sixth sense, for example, is unreliable. But equally, the assumption that medicine is a totally rational process is also wrong. Doctors may be reasonably smart, but they repeatedly fall into common and well-defined traps.

Further, Horton draws our attention to Groopman's advice that

> [p]hysicians can guard against these traps by heightening their sense of self-awareness and becoming conscious of their own feelings and emotions, responses, and choices. All too few doctors have this skill today. Indeed, a doctor's training can instill utterly contrary traits – confidence and certainty, in particular, which might close off an awareness of one's usually unconscious weaknesses. Instead, uncertainties should be acknowledged. Unveiling what we are unsure about would not only be more honest, it would also likely promote a degree of collaboration between patient and doctor that has hitherto been lacking.[213,214]

Developed nations: cutting costs – prioritising patients and resources?

In the light of the US research, and Horton's references to Groopman's analyses of medicine today, in a paradoxical sort of way, prioritising patients and resources to reduce costs may actually enhance the health of the general population – as in many cases 'minimising disease-causing factors' and fewer needless medical interventions could actually have salutary effects! This theme is carried forward in a recent interview with Mike Farrar, chief executive of the NHS Confederation, 'which represents most health service organisations'. Farrar echoes previous arguments, asserting that '[people] must be confronted with their "care footprint" to convince them to make better use of limited NHS resources, just as environmentalists have used carbon footprints'. Further, he advises that 'the care footprint should differentiate between "discretionary use" – which can be controlled by lifestyle choices – and "non-discretionary" requirements such as for accidents and inherited disease'.[227]

In the Western world, there appear to be few options in terms of the path we need to tread if we are to avoid, as Roy Porter observed, medical consumerism that may lead to 'a life exposed to degrading neglect as resources grow overstretched and politics turn mean',[221] as evidenced in recent tabloid headlines – 'Don't give out cancer drugs if it's used to extend life', 'Patients must be spared false hope', 'Hospitals are treating the elderly like slabs of meat' and 'Elderly neglect shocks foreign nurses'. In the longer run, the main quandary for healthcare decision-makers may very well be, as Porter predicted a decade ago, how best 'to redefine its limits even as it extends capacity'.[221]

Developing nations: key ingredients for success?

Porter's argument, while compelling in industrialised countries, is of course not the main concern of most 'developing' nations whose populations, according to the Human Development Index,[228] number about 85.4% (approximately 5.7 billion) of the world's 7 billion and potentially rising population. In developing countries – especially Africa – progress has been variable[12] and reaching the Millennium Development Goals,[11] in particular reducing child mortality, will be difficult to achieve by 2015, as discussed in Chapter 1.

As Cristobal and Worley[229] rightly point out, 'merely increasing the number of doctors will not necessarily improve health outcomes'. Indeed, the Ateneo de Zamboanga University School of Medicine 'in the southwest tip of the southernmost island of the Philippines', started in 1994, may show the way forward for other socio-economically disadvantaged countries. Here, 'in a spirit of volunteerism' local physicians 'developed and taught the curriculum without any salary'. Faculty were either employed by the health service or had their own private practice. Their efforts have definitely been rewarded, evidenced, for example, by the infant mortality rate. While in 1994 infant mortality rate was 75–80 per 1000 live births, by 2008 this figure had been reduced sharply to 8.2 per 1000 live births. Unlike many other countries, where 60%–80% doctors are trained and then move on,[78] 'more than 80% of the school's graduates are practising in the Zamboanga region'. The Zamboanga experience may have lessons for other developing nations and highlights the importance of several factors that need to come together for major change in healthcare and the quality of life of the population – in particular – 'the social accountability model of preferential local student selection, community-based medical education, and altruistic community engagement'.

In terms of medical education, there appear to be at least three constructive contributions that the developed nations can make to those less fortunate. First, as indicated in the Zamboanga experience, is not to interfere with what works well already at the local level. Second, to share these stories with others, as Lord Crisp advises,[127] who need to address similar challenges. At present, it appears that while increasing funds are spent on programmes (e.g. malaria, tuberculosis, AIDS), 'it is shortsighted that so little is spent on operational research, on learning what works in specific contexts and how best to engage communities to use the tools available'.[230] Third, to provide resources – technical advice and many mediated electronically – supporting those being trained in healthcare roles or advising on complex medical procedures.

Healthcare by 2020 and beyond: 'back to the future'?

Globally, healthcare is at a point where the inequalities 'between rich and poor, revealed by nineteenth-century statisticians, remain, while the disparities between the health standards of the First and Third worlds have blatantly increased'.[231] *The World Health Report 2008*[61] argued soundly for a return to primary healthcare basics, 'which promotes a holistic approach to health that makes prevention equally important as cure in a continuum of care that extends throughout the lifespan' with 'WHO estimates that better use of existing preventive measures (reducing) the global burden of disease by as much as 78%'. Considering the lack of resources worldwide, 'globalization of unhealthy lifestyles, rapid unplanned urbanization and the ageing population to support health care', Dr Margaret Chan, WHO director-general, posits that '[v]iewed against current trends, primary health care looks more and more like a smart way to get health development back on track'.[80] However, these changes will not happen automatically, as 'health systems will not naturally gravitate towards greater fairness and efficiency', as a consequence, says the WHO report, 'deliberate policy decisions are needed'.[80] And, it will be increasingly important that those who will be impacted by the changes in healthcare education need to 'own' the decisions and get involved in an 'action' culture (*see* Chapter 5 for discussion). The health education providers cannot afford the type of situation described by Professor William Tierney, director of the Centre for Higher Education Policy Analysis at the University of Southern California, several years ago:

> Too few individuals are involved, meetings are sporadic and ineffective, and the delineation of responsibilities has too easily been ceded to harried administrators who frequently feel overloaded with the complex decisions that need to be made.[232]

From academic centres to academic systems and longitudinal integrated rotations or clerkships

There are, of course, major transformations that could not possibly be left to ad hoc arrangements or which are relegated to 'harried administrators'. One of these is a fundamental reform or direction highlighted in *The Lancet* Commission report and relates to the recommendation of expanding 'academic centres' to 'academic systems', 'as a key process in the transformation of health professional education for a new century'. Proceeding along these lines would necessitate collaborative involvement of senior healthcare and other planners and policymakers on a national scale'.

As outlined in *The Lancet* report, '[a] long-standing problem in Brazil' – which is most likely also the situation in many other countries – 'has been the mismatch between professional education and the human resource requirements of the National Health System'. To tackle this issue, two ministries, Education and Health, 'launched a new partnership for reform', and '[a]ll academic institutions are reorienting their curriculum. The shift essentially involves re-directing training from hospitals to clinics and communities, to focus on prevention and social determinants, and to strengthen proactive, problem-based learning.' In Brazil, funding has been provided for '[m]ore than 500 courses, 9,000 fellowships, and the training in 14 health professions based in more than 80 institutions of higher education … in this partnership between two key ministries.'[56]

Complementing these core transitions and echoing innovations adopted in several ountries,[233] Professor Dr Marcelo Marcos Piva Demarzo, a specialist in family and community medicine, at the University of São Paulo, Brazil, reinforces the point that 'new curricula strategies are fundamental for the realisation of *The Lancet* Commission vision', and in his experience in Brazil, there are many benefits of 'increasing use of longitudinal integrated clerkships' and proposes the concept of a 'health-system-based clerkship'.[234]

> Ideally, a health-system-based clerkship would provide clinical medical training nested into a national health system, encompassing regional networks of primary care centres, outpatient clinics, and hospitals, with primary care as the clinical backbone that coordinates and longitudinally integrates scenarios, practices, and training. Such a programme could enhance meaningful interprofessional education for medical students, favouring continuity of training and care, patient and community-centredness, and social accountability.

This kind of pedagogic approach could cover the diversity and complexity of clinical experience and education expected for the new century's doctors in an 'academic system'.

Remote care requirements for NASA and community-based medicine

What may seem unusual but could potentially provide many advantages to community-based healthcare is the research undertaken by Dr Robert Marchbanks from the Neurological Physics Group at Southampton University Hospitals Trust and Dr Edward Good, a physician in neurological research at NASA's Johnson Space Center in Houston, Texas. Their investigations draw parallels 'between the remote care requirements for NASA and community/rural based medicine'. In their paper *Complex Neurological and Oto-neurological Remote Care: from space station to clinic*,[235] they demonstrate the appropriateness of applying similar 'health-care models of space-based medicine as for 2020 vision[236] community-based medicine and the common use of screening devices with telemedicine capabilities'. Considering both medical contexts, '[t]here is a requirement to diagnose and manage complex cases remotely and the need to empower on-site medical trained personnel to undertake the physiological measurements and decision-making', with 'the common aim of the need for hospitalisation – in both cases the issues are logistics, convenience and cost'.

Acknowledging the severe funding constraints across the globe, the researchers confirm the directions of international bodies and expert panels[56] and conclude that 'the present healthcare model is considered to be unsustainable under the 2020 vision' and that 'there is an increasing expectation that diagnostic assessments that are currently undertaken at the tertiary/specialist level should be undertaken at an earlier stage in the patient care pathways, and wherever possible, during primary assessment.' This shift 'is logistically better for the patient and their carers, will assist with earlier diagnosis and treatment, and is anticipated to reduce individual patient management costs at a time when overall healthcare costs are escalating'.[236]

Their '2020 vision' model – 'whether Earth or Space-based – recognises the requirement for specialist expertise (driven by innovation and not simply a medical consultant specialist with a video link) and sophisticated screening technology to be integrated at primary care level or remote space stations'. Finally, the researchers maintain that '[t]o ensure success there will be a need for collaborative partnerships between industry, universities and international government agencies including health services, departments of defence and homeland security, and space agencies such as NASA'. Calling 'for exemplary pilot studies for medical screening devices that have a telemedicine capability', the researchers' innovative thinking has the potential of influencing healthcare not only in the developed world but also, and perhaps most important, in those countries that have the greatest need.

Reducing costs, yet safer and more efficient treatment?

Referencing briefly Roger Bootle's[2] argument that we can learn much from countries like China and India, as there are a number of fields where they are starting to lead, it appears that medicine may very well be one of these. Nick Seddon, deputy director of the independent think tank Reform, recently observed open heart surgery at the Narayana Hrudayalaya cardiac hospital in Bangalore, India.[237] The American patient with a complex medical history had a valve replacement that was both risky and rare. The patient chose this hospital, as 'doctors there perform significantly better than most Western hospitals and patients are five times less likely to suffer from post-surgical complications'. The main reason for the hospital's excellent track record, according to Seddon, is that 'the doctors only deal with hearts', its specialist focus. In 2008, Narayana's 42 doctors 'performed more than 8,000 operations, a volume unheard of in the West, and waiting times less than a week' and 'at a tenth of the UK price'. Seddon notes that '[a]s volume and quality increase, costs also come down. Cited by Seddon, Dr Devi Shetty 'observed [w]e've looked at assembly lines, manufacturing plants, low-cost aviation and successful service industries and applied the lessons'. To achieve better patient outcomes at less cost, Seddon advises that the NHS needs to open up to these cutting-edge practices but this will mean doing things very differently. It also needs to focus on performance, hold doctors 'accountable for how money is spent, learn from other industries and be opened up to competition'. The Bangalore experience will likely influence needed changes in hospital services in many countries.

Atul Gawande, a surgeon and well-known author, in his book *Complications: a surgeon's notes on an imperfect science*,[238] reached similar conclusions. As an example, he notes that hernia repair 'takes about ninety minutes and might cost upward of four thousand dollars' and that the operation fails in about 10%–15% of the cases. He then references the Shouldice Hospital in Toronto, Ontario, Canada, 'where none of the statistics apply'. At Shouldice, hernia operations take about 30–45 minutes and 'their recurrence rate is an astonishing 1%. And the cost of an operation is about half of what it is elsewhere.' The secret of success, he concludes, 'is that at Shouldice the dozen surgeons do hernia operations and nothing else. … Each surgeon repairs between six hundred and eight hundred hernias a year – more than most general surgeons do in lifetime.' The other reason for their success, resonating with Horton's[213] review of Groopman's book,[214] is that 'all the repetition changes the way they think' and that '[w]ith repetition a lot of mental functioning becomes automatic and effortless, as when you drive a car to work'. On the other hand, '[n]ovel situations … usually require conscious thought and "workaround" solutions, which are slower to develop, more difficult to execute, and more prone to error'.

'What's past is prologue'

Revitalising medical education and training for the twenty-first century

Transforming medical education: seizing the moment

Borrowing a Shakespearian metaphor for the heading of the penultimate chapter, some may concur that we are entering a new era in medicine, medical education and healthcare generally. From a historical perspective the changes Western and Eastern societies are going through with regard to the global economy, climate change, energy shortages and lifestyle generally seem as profound today as the years from the 1890s to the 1940s, which ushered in the modern era.

While few major advancements in medicine and medical education took place up to the late nineteenth century, the twentieth century reversed years of delay, 'professional' bickering and strife and saw many achievements – although mainly in developed countries – despite major world conflicts, pandemics and recessions. This fast pace of change, accelerated largely through scientific research in the late nineteenth century, also proved to become the victim of its own success. Some of the deleterious side effects have included the emergence of diseases of affluence, over-reliance on hospital care and eventually expectation of the 'quick fix'. In Western societies, as health technology and care became centred in the hospital, community-based care became less important. Healthcare training programmes at both undergraduate and advanced levels reflect the biomedical model of disease and focus much more on cure than on prevention. With healthcare systems trying to respond to new demands (e.g. obesity and diabetes, other chronic conditions), with the expectation to apply the latest technological interventions, treatment has become more depersonalised and more costly. However, as argued in Chapter 1, healthcare has not necessarily become more equitable or effective even though in nations such as Britain a cardinal principle has been that as far as patient care is concerned everyone is equal. Variability of patient care has widened[108] and may reflect the availability of funding, often leading to a demoralised workforce. This scenario may describe healthcare in a number of countries, but it does not do justice to what is happening in less developed nations, some of which are just embarking on this medical journey, or others that wished they could.

Susan Greenfield in *Tomorrow's People*[4] may be speaking for many when she posits that society and individuals 'will have to make much more effort to comprehend what is happening, possible perspectives and take steps to prevent potential hazards'. Although '[t]he idea of everyone sitting down and talking is admirable … it is not a plausible solution'. She reiterates the need to 'work from the bottom up' in finding solutions to very complex problems and to chase the question: 'What single common factor might there be, what single issue is most important in our lives, which we wish to preserve at all costs?' In health and social care, it must surely be on the insistence of quality and safe care to ensure the well-being of patients and those requiring social care support. Her query may be an excellent starting point to bridge global visions and reforms relating to healthcare with local leadership and initiatives. Armed with a number of national and international reports and recommendations calling for change in this decade, policymakers are trying to respond to some of the issues, as well as others, outlined in this chapter introduction. And, in trying to locate areas where there may be obstacles to change, we may be reminded of the lead authors' conclusions in *Who's Got the Power? Transforming health systems for women and children*[7] (*see* Chapter 1 for discussion). Their main concern – the main reason why many of the Millennium Development Goals will not be achieved by 2015 – was the disconnect between developments and 'the broader economic and political forces'. This observation may also resonate with healthcare reforms. In the final analysis, making a positive difference to the lives of people 'is about the distribution of power and resources',[7] and getting the politicians and other stakeholders on side is perhaps one of the top priorities while 'seizing the moment'.

Factors underpinning long-term, highly successful organisations

Alex and David Bennet – both experts in knowledge management and organisational development – founded the Mountain Quest Institute in the United States – 'a research and learning center dedicated to working with individuals, groups and organizations to achieve growth, understanding and high performance in this age of change, uncertainty, complexity and the increasing anxiety resulting from change, uncertainty and complexity'.[239] In a comprehensive historical over-view of organisational evolution, they cite Collins and Porras's 6-year study of 18 companies that had outstanding performance over time periods between 50 and 200 years.[240] Their study, based on their research project at the Stanford University Graduate School of Business, sought to identify 'the fundamental factors creating such performance'. Building on Collins and Porras's results with other research, Alex and David Bennet identified the following factors 'as being representative of long-term, highly successful organisations':

- *Continuous striving to improve themselves and doing better tomorrow* than what they did today, always remaining sensitive to their customers and their environment.
- Not focusing on profitability alone, but *balancing their efforts to include employee quality of life, community relations, environmental concerns, customer satisfaction and stakeholder return.*
- A willingness to *take risks with an insistence that they be prudent* and an overall balanced risk portfolio. In general, they were financially conservative.
- A *strong feeling about their core ideology*, changing it seldom if ever. Their core values form a solid foundation and while each company's individual values were unique, once created they were not allowed to drift with the fashions of the day. This core value moulded their culture, and created a strong sense of identity.
- Relative to their employees, these companies demanded a *strong 'fit' with their culture and their standards.* Thus, employees either felt the organisation was a great place to work and flourished or they were most likely short-term. At the same time they were tolerant of individuals on the margins who experimented and tested for possibilities.

There is much to take away from these longitudinal studies. Alex and David Bennets' research helps to explain the deep-seated values identified by Professor Russell Mannion *et al.* in their study of NHS cultures outlined in Chapter 6.[174] Equally relevant, the Bennets' findings underscore how these values and beliefs are difficult to budge. Their five main conclusions also reinforce the importance of recognising 'employee quality of life' as well as customer/patient satisfaction. With the financial turmoil, these relationships are currently under strain in many health systems and may become more so as structural changes are accelerated, including refocusing healthcare from the hospital to the community and challenging the producer interests, in particular the medical establishment and eliminating needless and costly bureaucracy. Without these interventions, many have argued some health systems will 'atrophy and fail.' Perhaps the most important message, and one that may apply to today's state of medicine and medical education, is the criticality – including both healthcare organisations and educational institutions – of 'striving for self-improvement day in and day out and to invest in new technologies and new management methods, to take risks instead of lying back and remaining conservative. An eye should always be kept for the long term instead of the short term, even when it is hard to do so.'[241]

In summary, successful healthcare and academic providers tend to be ones that are sensitive to patient/client/learner needs – offering convenience, flexibility and quality of care and educational practice. They provide choice and anticipate patient/client/learner preferences and demand that responsibility rests with the person, not the system; they value staff commitment and service. These organisations are usually perceived externally and internally as 'reliable' and provide 'value-added' service and support. They also promote collaboration and the cross-pollination of ideas and value those who pay attention to detail; two examples of this are that elderly patients are well fed and looked after and that students have the opportunity to enhance their skills while developing teamwork, empathy and compassion.

Organisational reorientation: shifting the paradigm[138]

In *Evolution of Organizations: from bureaucracy to intelligent complex adaptive systems,*[239] the Bennets underscore that 'major opposition to new practices frequently comes from middle management's unwillingness to give up its prerogatives of decision-making and authority' and '[b]efore an organisation can adopt new practices … it must be willing to admit that its current practices are inadequate. This requires a paradigm shift and a willingness to adapt new assumptions in terms of how the business works and what must be done.'

Although, as discussed in Chapter 5, transformational change is problematic, it is vital that 'the seeds of positive attitudinal change are planted early' and to make 'reducing resistance to change a key part of this process and of institutionalisation'.[242] In this regard, Edgar Schein's conclusion seems particularly timely and pertinent: culture can be changed only when 'implicit and silent assumptions' are 'brought to the surface and confronted'.[173] This openness requires critical reflection on significant issues, which could in turn lead to 'perspective transformation'.[243]

Bolman and Deal[172] provide a 'human' explanation of why major change in any organisation, including healthcare education, often leads to conflict and the impact it may have on those affected by the change.

> Change usually benefits some people more than others: it creates winners and losers, which is bound to produce conflict. Change agents often underestimate

the opposition or drive conflict underground. Attention to the political dimensions of change implies recognising competing interests and creating arenas with rules, roles, and referees to provide conflicting individuals and groups with an opportunity to air and negotiate their differences.

Change also produces loss, particularly for those who are the targets rather than the initiators of change. Old patterns, familiar routines, and taken-for-granted meanings are all disrupted by organisational change. The deeper the loss, the more important it is to create rituals of transition – opportunities to both celebrate and mourn the past and help people evolve new structures of meaning.

These personal and professional adjustments are especially difficult to make in the current environment within which organisations must 'survive and thrive', and where 'Time accelerates. Distance shrinks. Networks explode. Interdependencies grow geometrically. Uncertainty dominates. Complexity overwhelms.'[244]

Expanding from local and national to global health systems

Considered collectively, these and other exemplars seem to be pointing to the path that healthcare education needs to take in order to respond constructively to the issues highlighted in several national studies, and, most recently, in the international *The Lancet*-commissioned report, which found 'fragmented, outdated, and static curricula that produce ill-equipped doctors, nurses, midwives, and public health professionals'.[56]

Nationally, as discussed in Chapters 3 and 4, high on the list of priorities must surely be the redesign of the medical curriculum – alongside other healthcare curricula – to ensure its cohesion, relevancy and vitality – underpinned, ideally, by sound educational philosophies that steer, guide and unite professional regulators, healthcare educators and learners.

Globally, interdependence 'underscores the ways in which various components interact with each other', and also involves three fundamental shifts:[56]
- from isolated to harmonised education and health systems
- from stand-alone institutions to networks, alliances and consortia
- from inward-looking institutional preoccupations to harnessing global flows of educational content, teaching resources and innovations.

Confirming a key enabling objective of *The Lancet* report, Gerald Keusch and colleagues examined institutional arrangements for malaria research. From their research,

[t]here is compelling evidence that long-term investments in education and training at many levels (e.g., national, provincial, district) can result in large payoffs for improved health. The global health system should prioritize additional investments in longer-term, multidisciplinary education and training for leadership in the complex public health, medical, management, economic, education, communications, and policy aspects of health systems, and in the functioning of health systems overall.[230]

Toward new curriculum models of healthcare education and training

According to *The Lancet* commissioners, the dominant approach to training health professionals is shown in Figure 9.1, whereby in the top horizontal diagram, each profession is trained separately or in 'closed' systems. In contrast, mirroring workplace practice, emerging models would concentrate much more on inter- and trans-professional teamwork (e.g. doctors, allied health professionals, administrators, managers).[56]

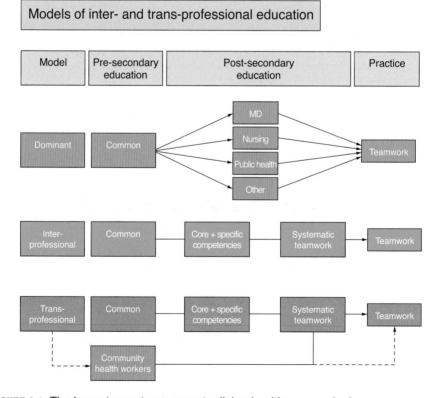

FIGURE 9.1 *The Lancet* report: reconceptualising healthcare curricula

As discussed in Chapter 4, applying this inter/trans-professional framework would first require determining healthcare competencies (non-clinical and clinical) that are common across the wide spectrum of professions in each of the years of learning engagement, recognising that lengths of programmes differ. Secondly, planners would need to identify areas of learning that are unique or specific to a particular profession and that essentially give the profession its main focus or professional identity.

Figure 9.2 is an attempt at illustrating how core (common) competencies and learning outcomes might be intertwined or meshed with profession-specific expectations in a 4-year programme with proportionally increasing collaborative learning and working in later clinical settings. Along with addressing issues of hierarchy, reformulating healthcare curricula along these lines would also address concerns relating to healthcare professionals working in 'silos'. One of the main concerns with current healthcare training and practice is simply that roles or units frequently appear to function independently, thereby increasing the possibility of compromising patient safety and the quality of care.

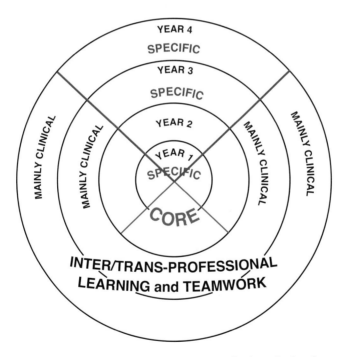

FIGURE 9.2 An inter/trans-professional healthcare curriculum design framework

The view that interprofessional and transprofessional teamworking may be an important factor in healthcare training is, according to a Scottish Council for Research in Education (SCRE) study,[245] driven by at least four factors:

1. Work practices that require members of different professions to work

together

2. A focus on the end user and the development of concepts of a 'seamless service' and joined-up policy
3. Increased demand from both potential and actual service users
4. A desire to ensure that public services are delivered efficiently, thus minimising duplication and waste.

Of these, perhaps the most fundamental and almost paradigmatic change that has occurred in the past few decades in most social, health and educational contexts has been the refocusing from the service supply side to service demand, the end user, in higher education, the student, and in health or social care, the patient and client, respectively. This reorientation is not new. In medical education, as far back as 1998 and a few years before, Sir Donald Irvine, then president of the GMC, noting that there were 'many important consequences of change', stated that 'now more than ever, the patient has come centre stage. The consumer is king'.[99] While the reasons for this transition may be obvious, they are not always clear to the suppliers, who usually have competing priorities – managing budgets, league tables, research, education, public perception, politics, to name only a few areas.

The importance of this mindshift cannot be overestimated, as it has implications for policy development, funding and patient care generally. As many will agree, and along with similar pressures felt in other nations, discussed in Chapter 1, UK healthcare is at a critical point with health inflation running at 7%, an ageing population, rise in chronic conditions and the need to save £20 billion by 2015 with demand for a 4 per cent improvement in productivity each year. Exacerbating the present situation is the call for improved services. As one example, Katherine Murphy, chief executive of the Patients Association[246] cited a press release from Niall Dickson, the chief executive of the GMC,[247] which reminded doctors that 'their care does not end with providing clinical treatment' and that 'they have a duty to take "prompt action"' whenever there are 'problems with basic care for patients who are unable to drink, feed or clean themselves'. Murphy further emphasised that '[d]octors should see a patient as a human and whatever their need they should be able to provide it'. Moreover, she noted '[i]t should be as much a doctor's responsibility as any other member of staff. Their duties go beyond clinical care and include dignity and respect. It's surprising that doctors need to be reminded.'[246]

The gap between good patient care, social client support and poor care appears to have widened since Sir Donald Irvine wrote his article, *Medicine beyond 2000: trust me I am (still) a doctor* in 1998, and many must be questioning where or how health and social care providers seemed to have lost their way or at least are under increasing public scrutiny. Two main arguments put forth in this book, and that are also reflected in national and international studies, are (1) the limitations or drawbacks of continuing 'uniprofessional' approaches in health and social care training, particularly with regard to doctors, nurses and social services and (2) the over-reliance on hospital or institutional care, when for most people community support – even at street level, as in parts of Germany – should be the preferred option for the future.

Addressing delegates at a United Nations high-level meeting on the prevention and management of non-communicable diseases, Eva Maria Ruiz de Castilla, member of the International Alliance of Patients' Organizations Governing Board, makes this point emphatically. Mirroring *The Lancet* report's major themes,[56] and while reminding delegates of the importance that their 'discussions will have on daily lives', she convincingly tells the delegates 'to keep the patient experience in mind':

> Too often, solutions are presented without talking to those most affected by them. But you cannot help someone, or provide a solution, if you do not know what the complete problem is, what it is like to 'walk in their shoes.' Involving communities in the decisions that affect them is not a luxury, but a must, if effective, relevant treatment and care is to be developed and delivered. Patient involvement and patient-centred healthcare therefore must be at the heart of health systems and goes hand in hand with a primary healthcare approach that recognises the interdependency and responsibility of all stakeholders to work together.[248]

Building teamwork, not 'team work'

However, as the authors of the SCRE report[245] conclude, 'putting people together in groups representing many disciplines does not necessarily guarantee the development of shared understanding'. They cite a study where nurse trainees shared lectures 'with medical students or students in training for professions allied to medicine who followed a common first year course with nurses'. The main finding was that the students 'did not appear to develop an enthusiastic approach to multidisciplinary working with other members of the health care team. Often they sat in segregated groups and expressed concerns about the lack of opportunities to consolidate their own sense of professional identity.'

From an outsider's point of view, there appear to be three main issues. First is the need to provide frequent informal socialising opportunities for these students before and during their courses. Second, the curriculum should ensure that students are able to learn and work together, under supervision, in realistic or patient-based (including simulations and use of mannequins) learning contexts where the students actually have the chance to engage with patients and one another. In the early years, working in small interprofessional groups, this activity could include interviewing patients about their experience of being a patient in home, institutional or hospital care. Shadowing other healthcare professionals and patients to get a better understanding of their roles and responsibilities could also be an important activity. Third, comparing their findings and reflecting on their experience could offer excellent opportunities for developing further understanding, respect and empathy.[88]

In clinical years, inter/trans-professional healthcare teams should be organised to work together on placements, in the community and hospitals, rural and urban. Individually, students should be encouraged to shadow each other in clinical and social care environments and discuss their experience afterwards with their peers and facilitators. The focus should always be on the patient or client and on how the team was supporting him or her, and what other interventions may be considered in consultation with the patient, family and the community. The SCRE observations confirm that lectures are far from suitable for achieving the aims of interprofessional education and indeed may reinforce stereotyping. A third consideration, as discussed earlier, is to review student selection criteria, providing a better balance between prerequisites in the sciences and social skills, especially empathy and compassion, which should be evidenced through prior experience. The healthcare profession needs people who truly care, who place more emphasis on nurture, rather than judging.

The preferred learning option, therefore, is through collaborative (inter/trans-professional) practice that leads, as Kolb's learning cycle[249] suggests (*see* Figure 9.3), from an actual patient or client experience to reflection, and to theorising about what went well, what didn't, and ways to improve and applying and making changes the next time. At present, students are often exposed to theory

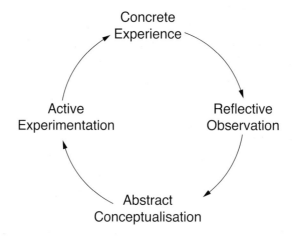

FIGURE 9.3 Kolb's learning cycle

or abstract conceptualisation (often in large group lectures) with delays (days and sometimes weeks) – occurring in terms of practical application, with very little reflection in and on practice,[136] and rare patient or interdisciplinary input.

The key questions concern matching competency expectations with appropriate learning experiences and placing students into situations where they can acquire greater understanding of each other's roles by actually 'doing' healthcare rather than 'shop talk'. Ann Smith and John Stephens advocated using 'critical incidents as a means of learning, which uncovered emotional factors as well as perceptions, values and assumptions'. An example of such an approach would be asking students to 'consider an incident from clinical practice that caused them to be puzzled, angry, proud or sad' and to 'think about the questions this incident raises regarding the relationship between theory and practice'.[250]

Responding to *The Lancet* Commission report, students support 'team-based education to break down the silos'[251] and have actually been in the vanguard in establishing an international forum that includes medicine, nursing, pharmacy and allied health professions. Their annual World Healthcare student symposia aim to encourage greater understanding of different professions and to identify the best ways of effective and fruitful collaboration. The students' final plea is '[w]hat students try to teach themselves through laborious but successful efforts should not be neglected by their educational institutions'. Nor, it may be argued, should these initiatives of shared learning be undermined by 'professional territoriality' or 'profession ethnocentrism derived from professional identity and socialisation'.

Achieving the aims of 'working together' will not happen by chance and requires good curriculum design as well as putting adult learning theory[252] – which is learner- not content-centred – into effective practice, in particular the need for active learning engagements rather than endless hours of lectures, followed often by multiple-choice tests. It also necessitates a combination of 'committed individuals, a common sense of purpose, clarity in team roles and explicit support from the host organisation'[245] along with financial investment and endorsement by health regulators, and support from the professional bodies that may need to debate how best to avert or 'nip in the bud' entrenched attitudes that may – as in previous centuries – reinforce traditional professional hierarchies and practices.

From a student development perspective that seeks to strengthen interprofessional teamwork, it is crucial that more faculty develop the expertise to facilitate interprofessional education and for organisations to make a purposeful effort to retrain faculty as interprofessional educators. Role modelling can be a powerful motivator to encourage students from diverse healthcare professions to collaborate effectively in the work environment.

In a very informative Association of Medical Educators in Europe (AMEE) guide, *Theoretical Insights into Interprofessional Education*, Dr Sarah Hean and colleagues advocate 'the need for theory in the development and practice of inter-professional education'. The guide provides many examples of good practice and 'highlights a range of theories that can be applied to interprofessional education', in particular those supporting the social dimension of interprofessional learning, while also exploring the practical application of these theories.[253]

Future technological advances and healthcare

While prognostications may be common, their value is doubtful; for example, it is said that Lord Kelvin, president of Britain's Royal Society, predicted in the 1890s that X-rays will prove to be a hoax, and Tom Watson's doubtful prediction, as chair of IBM's Board in 1943, 'I think there is a world market of maybe five computers.' Former president of the Institute for the Future Ian Morrison identified several widespread mistakes of predicting the future. One of his observations, which may be useful to remember when implementing change in medical education, is the tendency of 'overestimating the effect of short-term change and underestimating the effect of long term change'.[254] Richard Klausner, director of the US National Cancer Institute, says just about the same thing but adds, 'We're not that bad at predicting things that might be part of the future, but we're really bad at predicting the timing and kinetics and path to them.'[5]

Placing much more faith than Dr Jerome Groopman[214] in the use of technology in patient care, and speculating about the future, Leroy Hood, affiliate professor of immunology and president of the Institute for Systems Biology, suggests that by 2018, patients will be able to carry out a medical home check-up using a handheld device, which can make as many as 2000 different measurements, pinprick a finger, draw off a fraction of blood and send the data to a distant computer for analysis.[255] Fewer young patients will be seen by their doctors, as their conditions will be detected early by their 'biosensors allowing GPs to nip diseases in the bud'. By 2020 we may be able to grow complete heart replacements for use in transplants. Others believe that a combination of stem cell research, synthetic genomics, nanotechnology and other breakthroughs will lead to cures for a wide range of illnesses as early as 2030. These include AIDS/HIV, the majority of cancers, motor neurone disease, arthritis and diabetes and (perhaps in the realm of sci-fi?) that we will be even able to download the human brain by 2030.[256] At about the same time, with increasing life expectancy, some suggest that most wards will be filled with centenarians, whereas those in their 70s, 80s and 90s remain healthy, independent and active members of the community.[257] According to archaeologist and historian Ian Morris from Stanford, it is probable that at some point in this century (perhaps 2080s?) there will be a merging of human beings and machine, and we can expect 'new ways of living, fighting, working, thinking and loving, new ways of being born, growing old, and dying'.[3] An important dimension of monitoring and sharing human progress this century, which should be made easier through technological inventiveness, relates to increasingly 'making arrangements for sharing knowledge of successful system strengthening', as advocated by Lord Crisp.[258]

Finally, as Professor Alejandro R Jadad and Murray W Enkin, Emeritus Professor, observe in their *BMJ* article 'Computers: transcending our limits?'[259] we may need to be mindful that while '[e]xtrapolations of 20th century trends into 21st century visions are not optimistic, … extrapolation does not acknowledge the complexity of evolution. … A more exciting scenario may be unfolding, in which the future is not predetermined by immutable forces but shaped by our values, our interactions, and our will to survive as autonomously as possible against all odds.'

Further, the authors hypothesise that '[t]he 21st century computer age gives us the opportunity to create a "noosphere," a true planetary thinking network with individual but interdependent humans as its nodes. The exponential development of wireless networks, mobile computing tools, and the internet may already be giving us a glimpse of a future in which we could work as "humanodes" in a true global superorganism.'

Several years ago, in a refreshing and imaginative essay entitled, 'What will doctors be doing by 2050?'[257] a first-year medical student provided her personal glimpse of being a doctor mid twenty-first century. Few will wish to disagree with her optimistic and cheerful outlook, which evidently follows Professors Jadad and Enkin's train of thought.

> 12:30 p.m.
> Technological advances and the expansion and refinement of biological understanding have had a substantial impact on what doctors can now do for their patients. Doctors must be aware of the minefield of Methics. Today, I am chairing an e-debate on Methics with Dr. Wong, a fertility expert from China, and Dr. Dubois from France. The debate will be broadcast to students all over the world (thank goodness for autotranslaters)! E-lectures are a great educational tool, allowing us to pool international knowledge and thought. Doctors today truly work in an international environment: sharing research, uniting in the fight against illness and breaking down the long-standing barriers between orthodox and complementary medicine. Embryo screening for personality, intelligence, gender and looks still remain hot ethical and legal issues. Our lecture also explores the moral problems raised by the growth of non-health related medicine. Cosmetic surgery has rocketed in popularity, encouraged by targeted personalised advertising.[257]

Managing the change process

At the launch of *The Lancet*-commissioned report, *Health Professionals for a New Century: transforming education to strengthen health systems in an interdependent world*,[56] members of the Strategies for Dissemination panel concluded that the report and its recommendations needed to be spread widely, using 'the convening power of other global initiatives and partnerships' and taking 'advantage of networking opportunities and social mobilisation models'. Given the potential global impact of the Commission's report, '[e]veryone needs to spread the message and find allies among colleagues, young professionals and leadership; every region or country needs its own champion for change'.[260]

There are, of course, the next stages to consider – one of the main purposes of this book – and that is making it all happen. Overall, change outcomes proposed by national and international panels or commissions, seeking to improve healthcare education, have two common aims: first, to increase effectiveness – that is, to ensure the safety and quality of care for the patients; second, to enhance efficiency – that is, to reduce the cost for the organisation or, essentially, to do more with less.

However, it may be important to remind ourselves that achieving these ends, as outlined in Chapter 5, requires 'the commitment of individuals who see the change as a highly personal experience, entailing their own developmental growth and skills.[261] Referencing William Bridges' seminal book *Managing Transitions: making the most of change*,[262] Alexandra Katseva, a senior systems consultant, notes his distinction between 'change' and 'transition', observing (*see* Figure 9.4), that the former is situational and leads to an event or an invention – new teams, new roles – whereas 'people's adoption and acceptance of new processes is psychological – a personal transition – that people must go through to accept the change'.[263]

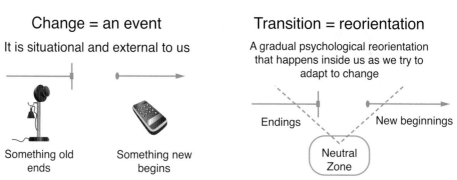

FIGURE 9.4 Change management versus psychological transition

Reminiscent of Bolman and Deal's organisational change model,[172] referenced previously, Figure 9.5 suggests that people essentially proceed through three phases when confronted with a major change. Each of these, Bridges notes, needs to be carefully managed.[262]

1. Ending, Losing, Letting Go
2. The Neutral Zone
3. The New Beginning

In Figure 9.4, the x-axis illustrates time while the y-axis indicates proportionality in terms of management activity required to support the change.

Managing endings

Bridges argues that 'it isn't the changes that do you in, it's the transitions'. In other words, 'it is the personal and psychological side of change related to people's transitions that is difficult to manage rather than the explicit program of planned activity such as installing new computers or putting in place new incentive programs or reorganising a workforce'.[262] Further, Bridges asserts that because transition is a process by which people 'unplug from an old world and plug into a new world', transition is a process that starts with an ending – letting go of the old reality – and ends with a beginning. Staff, he posits, must be allowed to come to terms with their own personal 'endings' and the change-makers need to be open about their losses and how things will be different; it is also important to accept sympathetically the reality and importance of their losses; as emotions

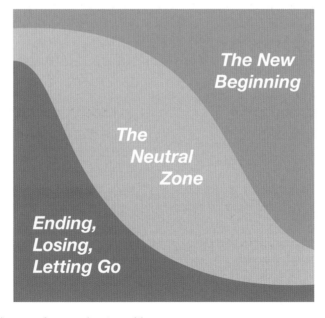

FIGURE 9.5 Phases of managing transitions

surface, overreaction is normal and it is important for policy- or change-makers to expect and accept signs of grieving as well as feelings of anger, anxiety, sadness and disorientation recalling Bolman and Deals' similar concerns while contrasting 'winners' and 'losers' in any major change initiative.[172] It is also vital to keep people up to date about what is happening and why, if possible 'to compensate for losses' and to treat the past with respect. One of the main reasons changes fail is that endings are poorly managed and the key step for transition teams is not to understand the destination but how to get people to convince people 'to leave the old situation behind'.

Managing the 'neutral' zone

After people have let go of the past, they enter what Bridges calls 'the neutral zone'. The neutral zone is really a transition – 'a nowhere between two some-where's … while you are in it, forward motion seems to stop while you hang suspended between *was* and *will be*'. Here people will feel insecure and anxious, as the old way has gone and the new way does not yet feel right. The neutral zone is a phase that offers both risk and opportunity. Risk in the sense that anxiety rises, motivation decreases and productivity may fall, as discussed in Chapter 8. People may get confused between the old way and the new and polarise. It is important at this stage to try to protect staff from unexpected or unrelated changes and to ensure that new policies or procedures are put into place when needed (e.g. new policy on job descriptions, management structures). Bridges feels that the neutral zone is the best time for creativity and renewal, when innovation is most possible and when a new spirit of entrepreneurship can take hold rather than do what you are told. It is a time when people and systems 'unfreeze' from the old systems and have not yet frozen back into the new systems. It is a time when there is vast opportunity to identify and realise changes and find new ways of doing things. During this phase staff go through an inner 'sorting' process as they become more familiar with the new way. Bridges gives a number of mechanisms for this phase, including creating temporary support systems and short-term goals and redefinition of the activity in the neutral zone in terms of more familiar activity or metaphors.

Launching a new beginning

Bridges differentiates between 'starts' and 'beginnings'. A start occurs when people start doing new things, when they start enacting the changes. A 'beginning' cannot be forced or made to happen and only occurs when the personal psychological and behavioural change takes place and people assume new behaviours and identities or after they are prepared to make the necessary emotional commitment to do things the new way. Beginnings therefore involve new understandings, new values, new attitudes and – most of all – new identities.

Bridges encourages leaders to think along the lines of the 4 Ps: purpose, picture, plan and part to play. With regard to purpose, leaders need to explain clearly the rationale behind the new beginning, answering the question 'why are we doing this?' In some cases it is more important to sell the problems rather than the solutions. Clichés or jargon should be avoided. It is also important to translate abstract understandings into concrete reality – something people 'can see in their imaginations'. Visual aids may help in doing so. Further, it is vital to develop a plan for the transition, one that is more person-oriented and identifies when people will receive the information, training and support needed to make the transition. Perhaps, most importantly, people need to see their role and their relationship to others in the new order.

When the change is not well received, Bridges highlights that it is best to introduce change as one package, that is, not to break it down into smaller changes, and not to make threats and to take time to explain the changes very carefully, preferably in written memos rather than e-mails. Appointing a change manager and well-planned training seminars can also be productive if seen as part of a larger effort. Bridges also advises that it is very important to identify specifically the behaviours or attitudes that must stop and those that must start and to talk to individuals and ask what problems they are having and to hold regular meetings. Finding larger patterns that rationalise all the changes, rebuilding trust, healing old wounds and keep selling problems are key ways of dealing with non-stop change, Bridges argues.

A possible shortcoming of Bridges's book, as noted by Dr Lauchlan Mackinnon, an Australian organisational development consultant, is that while his 'framework is full of insights and remains a highly useful framework for conceptualising and managing change', it does not discuss 'the sociological and cultural dimensions of change for an organisation', as '[m]ajor change typically impacts not only individual people but also cultural shared values, behaviours, and collective identity'.[264]

Another lens through which to examine change and transitions is through Everett Rogers's 'diffusion of innovation' theory that tries to explain how, why and at what rate new ideas and technology spread through cultures, in a way complementing Bridges's work.

Rogers's innovation adoption curve[265] (*see* Figure 9.6) estimates that in every group there are only about 2.5% Innovators and only about 13.5% Early Adopters or potential leaders, who have the capacity to lead and propel the change initiative. It will largely depend on the ingenuity and skill of these enthusiasts to try to get about 34% of the staff on board who are the Early Majority, who tend to be cautious and deliberate about deciding to adopt an innovation. It may take a lot longer to secure the support of an equal number of about 34% who comprise the Late Majority and who are 'set in their ways'. However, with the right levers many of these may be swayed as well. The remaining 17% are the Laggards or resisters – suspicious and generally opposed to new ideas, but some of these may too be won over when they observe that initiatives are making a positive difference in the work environment or when they are provided with new ideas to explore.

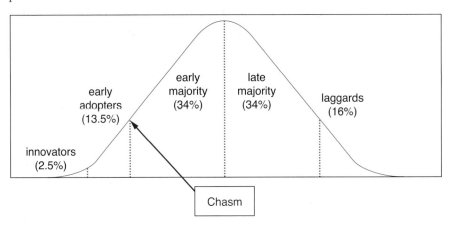

FIGURE 9.6 The diffusion of change[265]

Rogers advises that there may be some simple ways of securing individual and group level change, with Innovators and Early Adopters requiring almost no encouragement, as they are ready to act on the change or innovation. The Early Majority could benefit from showing them a working example. With the Late Majority there is a need to prove that the change is beneficial and with Laggards there may be a need to 'change the rules!' While Rogers's normal curve may be fairly accurate in terms of the types of responses certain groups may make to major change initiatives, his theory may not go far enough in terms of taking into consideration the psychological journey that Bridges talks about.

Bridges would probably agree that the adoption gap – the chasm – lies between the Early Adopters and the Early Majority or the far edge of the 'neutral zone' and the near edge of 'The Beginning', and engaging these individuals needs to be a top priority as the transition process progresses. Some of the change approaches introduced in Chapter 5 could be instrumental in this regard, particularly the Change Matrix and the interactional leadership processes.

Juxtaposing Bridges's transition model with Rogers's theory of diffusion of innovation, we might find that the Innovators and Early Majority would spend the least time in the Ending phase, while the Late Majority spend slightly more and the Laggards may never psychologically leave the old ways. The same time pattern may play out with the 'neutral' or transition phase. It is here that the Late Majority might find their space and make their most creative contributions to the organisation – hence the bulge in the middle of this phase. If they can demonstrate or role model that the new way is better than the old, then the probability of the Late Majority supporting the change increases considerably. The New Beginning may then gather momentum and the change may feel 'normalised' or, that is, the way we do things around here; that is part of who we are: our identity.

A final approach to change that could readily be integrated into and contribute to previous change models identified in Chapter 5 and in this chapter is the Concerns-Based Adoption Model (CBAM).[266] Its uniqueness lies in that it not only focuses on the stages (*see* Figure 9.7) that people go through when faced with a major change – endings, transitioning, new beginnings – but also seeks to support or answer the types of questions people generally have while proceeding through various developmental stages, which move from the inner 'self' to the external 'task' to 'impact' on the wider environment. An assumption is that individuals may benefit from different types of interventions at various stages of concern and that leaders should take these into consideration when planning and managing change. Resonating with Bridges, the CBAM approach assumes that change (transition?) is a process and that there are incremental steps or 'natural, predictable stages of concern that individuals go through as they encounter change, new experiences and new demands'.[266]

> The model holds that people considering and experiencing change evolve in the kinds of questions people typically ask and in their use whatever the change is. In general, early questions are more self-oriented: What is it? and how will it affect me?

Later, when these have been

> resolved, questions emerge that are more task-oriented: How do I do it? How can I use these materials efficiently? How can I organise myself? And why is it taking so much time? Finally, when self- and task-concerns are largely resolved, then the individual can focus on impact. Educators ask: Is this change working for students? and Is there something that will work even better.[267]

These phases – self, task, impact – have considerable implications for project management and professional development, as '[f]irst they point out the importance of attending to where people are and addressing the questions they are asking when they are asking them' rather than the usual 'how to do it' questions; and second, 'the model suggests the importance of paying attention to implementation for several years, because it takes at least three years for early concerns to be resolved, and later ones to emerge.' Moreover, the concerns from managers, policymakers, professional bodies and others will also need to be addressed, in particular responding to the question, 'How will it affect me?' As Susan Loucks-Horsely reminds us '[t]he strength of the of the concerns model is in its reminder to pay attention to individuals and their various needs for information, assistance, and moral support'.[267]

It is probable that most of the concerns and questions will come from the Early and Late Majority, with greatest resistance from the latter cohort. Fundamentally, 'the extent to which people are more or less resistant, indifferent, or likely to lend support to change is affected by how they perceive the change affecting them. Reasons for resisting change have been studied and include:[268]

- loss of control
- too much uncertainty
- surprise
- confusion
- loss of face
- concerns about competence in a new context
- increased workload
- change fatigue
- the view that costs outweigh benefits
- past resentments.

Planners and decision-makers attempting to introduce transformative change in healthcare obviously need to be prepared to address these types of concerns at individual and group levels. However, the unifying thread that should keep the discussions on track needs to be the welfare of the patients in times of great uncertainty in all walks of life.

As we have seen in Chapter 5 and in Bridges's 'transition' as well as Rogers's 'diffusion of innovation' models, managing people through a change effort is as important as the project itself. Both authors would likely agree that successful change requires: 'the presence of identifiable enthusiasts – boundary-spanning individuals'[269] for making the change (Innovators and Early Adopters); 'conducive power relationships' (i.e. lack of conflict with national policies or professional opinion); adaptability to local conditions;[56] and 'a general perception that the innovation meets current needs along with minimal requirements for extra resources'.[270] In summary, while individuals have different attitudes to change, most 'want their jobs to be rewarding, secure, interesting and familiar. And, when faced with new roles and responsibilities resulting from a change effort, a likely first reaction will be negative and resistant.'[271] The previous models would suggest that there may be better alternatives to minimising the strength of this resistance.

The CBAM can also be useful in identifying approaches to change (*see* Figure 9.7), thereby propelling initiatives. Crucial for getting people on side is addressing personal concerns, possibly drawing on the interactional leadership framework discussed in Chapter 5. Listening to and focusing on the issues

Stages of Concern   **Interventions**

I	VI	Refocusing	How can we make it better? What needs to be done now?
M			
P	V	Collaboration	Share ideas with others Have others come to visit Present new ideas, projects at a conference
A			
C	IV	Consequence	Share sessions – show what works for you Survey teachers, students Pre and post data sharing Examining test scores Identify ways to measure impact (is it working?) Let her/him share success stories with you
T			
T	III	Management	Help with planning Help develop timelines Help organise committees Show you can organise to accomplish the same task Share time management techniques
A			
S			
K			
	II	Personal	Build trust relationships Offer moral support, confidence building Accept feelings and try to direct towards positive action Visit a site where innovation is being used to see it in action
S			
E	I	Informational	Clarify information (avoids fears about 'grapevine' information)
L			
F	0	Awareness	Provide printed materials to read Orientation session/workshop Videotape of programme in action Pair 'those who know' with 'those who do not'

FIGURE 9.7 Stages of concern and interventions[266]

identified and exploring how to resolve them together openly as equals seem to be central to good leadership. Emotions frequently override reason.

As shown in Figure 9.7, the CBAM is also a useful way of measuring levels of use or application of progress in terms of project outcomes.

Colleagues and I drew on the CBAM process in Canada with numerous projects. One of these related to implementing a telecommunication and information technology project at Mohawk College of Applied Arts and Technology, a large community college in Ontario, Canada at that time registering c. 10 000 full-time and c. 65 000 part-time students in a catchment area that served c. 375 000 residents. A key challenge facing the college was how to increase access by learners in existing and new full and part-time programmes and improving accessibility for adult learners. Another concerned identifying new revenue streams.

Funded by the provincial government,[272] the main purpose of the project was to broaden staff understanding of two telecommunications media: videoconferencing and telecourse delivery, as part of a distance learning strategy, by establishing provisional systems or opportunities. Applying the CBAM framework, we decided that part of the 'self' and 'task' concerns might best be addressed through the careful orchestration of a seminar series conducted by credible experts in open and distance learning. The overall aim of the series was 'to encourage staff to develop a positive view towards the use of telecourses which could then lead to a willingness to try out certain aspects'. At the conclusion of the eight-part series, which drew on expertise from the United States and Canada, including actual reviews of existing telecourses, and attended by a cross-section of staff members, all of whom had attended several of the previous seminars, and some of whom had also participated in site visits, participants were asked to identify barriers that they felt prevented the college from becoming more involved in full-time as well as part-time programming. In the main, issues could be grouped under three main categories: *teaching-related concerns* – holding on to traditional values with regard to teaching practices, job security, and incentives or motivation to change; *technical-related concerns* – fear of technology, lack of technology; and *organisational/financial concerns*, in particular relating to the cost of new support services.

Use of the CBAM was successful. Not only did the approach identify key issues that mattered to the staff and students, but it also found solutions to some of their basic reservations. At that time – the mid 1990s – the college did not make much use of distance learning or telecourses, but now it offers '550 courses, more than 40 Certificates and two Diploma programmes'. It appears that stages V (Collaboration – for example, sharing ideas with others) and VI Refocusing, that is, 'how can we make it better?' of the Concerns-based Adoption Model have been reached.

In retrospect, there were possibly eight factors that made the project viable initially and that encouraged proceeding with the initiative after the 'seed' funds were exhausted:

- a demonstrated (specific data) need (e.g. surveys and focus groups) for enhancing adult learner-centred education
- corporate strategic planning and investment and 'one-off' seed funds
- sensitivity to the concerns of all those who would be impacted by new innovative practices
- involvement of the communities and groups in market research
- use of external consultants who had direct experience of the innovation and drawing on concrete examples (e.g. telecourses, videoconferences)
- managing the change process in such a way in order to provide sufficient time to debate the implications of the change initiatives and to find compromise solutions

- formation of small interest groups with credible 'champions' assuming leadership roles and cross-pollination of ideas
- starting with a few successes and incrementally building outreach connections.

While this 'evolutionary' approach seems ideal, present challenges facing healthcare – quality of patient care and safety in the midst of severe financial constraints – may no longer allow such luxury. The present climate – and likely continuing in the foreseeable future – may precipitate a re-evaluation of resourcing and determining ideal and actual timespans for implementing transformative change in medical/healthcare education.

10

Facing limitations and challenges

Broadening the field of medicine and medical education in the twenty-first century

Human population growth and global carrying capacity

As confirmed throughout this text, it is clear that the healthcare needs and issues in the industrialised nations differ sharply from those in the developing world. While in the former many illnesses result from affluence, in many developing nations, especially in sub-Saharan Africa and southeast Asia, the central causation of poor health is poverty affecting approximately 1.6 billion people – more than one in seven of the total world population. The variance in the numbers affected should be a stark reminder of the inequity and urgency of addressing the problems, with approximately 5.7 billion people in poor countries with low or no income and approximately 1.3 billion people in high-income nations.

At a recent University College London and Leverhulme Trust symposium on human population growth and global carrying capacity,[273] several important messages emerged that should give cause for reflection and concern:

- The global population, doubling since 1967, and now at approximately 7 billion, will grow to about 8 billion by 2025, 9 billion by 2043, 10 billion by 2083 and 18 billion by 2100, if fertility and child mortality rates remain constant.
- Between now and 2030, demand for food will increase by 40%, and demand for energy and water will increase by 30%.

It is alarming and paradoxical that in developed countries about 50% of all food is discarded after purchase – reminding us of Mahatma Gandhi's observation that 'the world has enough for everyone's need, but not for everyone's greed' – and that 'in developing counties 50% is wasted before purchase because of pest infestation, poor storage'.[273]

Without question, global increases in population and consumption are leading 'to severe and negative impacts on health and well-being'. Further, the symposium organisers conclude that 'the most significant driver behind the world's environmental problems relates to 'unsustainable and inequitable patterns of consumption'. Moreover, '[s]ocial inequities, including wealth, consumption, gender and health inequities', are crucial 'as they are both the causes and consequences of unsustainable consumption and population growth and present major social and moral issues'. Echoing concerns from the 2005 study *Who's Got the Power? Transforming health systems for women and children,*[7] introduced in Chapter 1, while family planning is a crucial priority, 'there is insufficient funding to ensure universal access to sexual and reproductive health service'.

The 300 people from 33 countries who attended the University College London and Leverhulme Trust symposium, which was also linked to the satellite meeting of 100 delegates in Nairobi, Kenya, hosted by the African Institute for Development, in partnership with the Kenyan government, reached consensus on five key areas to address these challenges:

1. '[W]omen and their needs must be at the centre of population-related debates and interventions'.
2. Family planning must be free from coercion and 'part of comprehensive, reproductive and sexual health programmes that protect and respect human rights'.
3. 'Engaging with young people in the global South', meeting their needs for health and education and 'seizing opportunities' to realise 'the demographic dividend'.
4. Recognising that '[c]ountries of the developing South are increasingly identifying the need to address unsustainable rates of population growth' as well as 'pressure on resources'.
5. 'Technology and innovation have great potential to contribute to a green economy, sustainable agriculture and an overall sustainable development path'.

In a follow-up meeting, the 2011 experts, who attended the University College London and Leverhulme Trust symposium, acknowledged that much more needed to be done in terms of 'advocacy, public policy engagement and collaboration'. However, the question remains whether anything has really changed since 2005. Are the deeper structural issues still with us today or, given the global downturn, have they been made worse? That is, to what extent is there still a delinking of 'mainstream development practice ... from the broader economic and political forces that have generated a level of inequity, exclusion, divisiveness'? And, if the situation remains unchanged, how can this 'disconnect' be finally resolved?

As these concerns impact directly on the quality of life of all individuals – living generally in poor communities, perhaps community leaders from a cross-section of society (e.g. government, education, medical, religious) need to make more of a concerted effort to meet the huge daily challenges faced by about one in seven people in the world. With over 90 children of every 1000 dying before age five in the developing world, ranging from as low as 2.6 in Singapore to c. 180 in Angola, for many, it appears, that time is fast running out.

Sir David Attenborough, in the President's 'People and Planet' address to the Royal Society of Arts and Commerce, confirmed that the problems of population growth and consumption are not 'confined to the so-called "developing world"'.[274] According to Food and Agriculture Organisation figures, over 19 million people in the developed nations are also malnourished. One of the main reasons for this rise – and one that will likely escalate – is population growth. For example, 'unlike Europe, the US population is growing fast – from 200 million in 1970, to over 310 million today [2011] and a projected 420 million in 2050'. The ones who suffer the most are the children, where it is estimated that in the United States alone, 3.5 million children under the age of 5 are 'on the verge of going hungry' each day. However, the problem does not appear to be a lack of food but rather not taking advantage of systems that exist (e.g. the US food stamp programme). Poor health literacy, discussed in Chapter 1, could well be a major contributor to malnutrition in developed nations. Another cause is rapid urbanisation, as Sir Attenborough points out: 'By 2030, 5 billion people (over 60 per cent of the world's population) are expected to live in towns and cities. And while urban settlements have great potential to enrich life, the speed of their growth has led to immense environmental problems. Some 600 million city dwellers are today without adequate shelter and over 400 million do not have access to the simplest latrines.'

Finding solutions to emerging needs and problems

Professor David Wooton,[171] reflecting on medicine in past centuries, observes that only in the last century have we seen 'the emergence of a world in which medical knowledge established a positive feedback loop with medical therapy: progress in knowledge led to progress in therapy, which led to more investment in research'. Further, he argues what is holding doctors back from further progress is not 'economic self-interest' but 'the cultural identity of the medical profession, an identity transmitted through the texts of Hippocrates and Galen, and symbolised by the leech, the lancet and the tourniquet'. In his view '[w]hat held doctors captive was an imaginary world of their own creation, and the history of medicine may end as a history of science, but it needs to begin as a history of the medical imagination.' It is conceivable that *The Lancet* Commission report[56] as well as other international or national reports that are calling for fundamental changes in how medical education is enacted, might become the catalysts for the release of this 'imagination'. The main obstacles to achieving this transformation, however, may be the vested interests which 'protect their status as powerholders so tenaciously.'[276] As this book affirms, solutions to twenty-first century healthcare practices and medical education will not be easily found in previous century thinking, and, as Einstein is believed to have said, 'No *problem* can be solved from the *same* level of consciousness that created it.'

Given prevailing and disturbing realities in the developed and developing world, where many of the social, economic and health concerns – some of which have been identified in this book – are pressing for urgent reform, Professor Wooton's main conclusion may be accurate. To respond to the imbalances, inequities and unsettling lifestyle trends, what is needed now are creative or inventive, some would say 'outside-of-the-square', solutions to very basic human problems: how do we feed the world's hungry? What can we do about rising levels of obesity? How can prevention of disease become more central to healthcare rather than cure? How can we ensure that our children remain compassionate and empathetic and that the elderly are cared for with respect and dignity? And, how can we provide hope for those who have none? Everyone is a stakeholder in this global quest for answers, and there can be no doubt that bold and courageous leadership must find the way.[56]

Although the issues are dissimilar, there is a common thread that weaves through both the developed and developing worlds, as Michele Barry, senior associate dean for global health at Stanford School of Medicine, points out. In her view, the '[t]raditional approaches in medicine and public health are coming up against their limitations' and 'broadening the field of medicine to include new disciplines and sectors is critical'.[275]

For example, in the developed world, the urgent need for collective action – health, social, education, media – on a number of fronts is brought to a head by Baroness Greenfield, who is professor of pharmacology at Oxford University. In her recent book, *You and Me: the neuroscience of identity*,[276] she identifies a potential issue that may be ultimate victim of poor lifestyle choices – the human brain in the twenty-first century and how it will evolve. Citing several studies – one that 'addicts with an average age of 27 are spending on average 80 hours a week on online gaming', and another where UK 'children between their tenth and eleventh birthdays, spend on average 900 hours in class, 1,277 hours with their family and 1,934 hours in front of a screen' – she asserts that '[p]rolonged and frequent video gaming, surfing and social networking cannot fail to have an effect on the mental state of a species whose most basic and valuable talent is a highly sensitive adaptability in which it is placed'.

One consequence that might have huge implications for the healthcare professions is based on a study of '1,400 US college students [which] showed a decline in empathy over the past 30 years, with a particularly sharp drop in the past decade'. According to Professor Greenfield, '[s]creen-based violence has been associated with lower empathy; while repeated exposure to violent video games in turn increases aggressive behaviour via changes in personality factors associated with desensitisation'. In addition, she identifies a common factor between various states, such as 'gambling, eating, schizophrenia – and indeed being a child', and concludes that '[i]n all cases, the press of the senses, the here-and-now environment, is unusually paramount'. While the twenty-first century is making major advances technologically, there is the danger that, as Baroness Greenfield points out, 'constant exposure to a literal world, devoid of metaphor and abstract concepts' could lead to the user's brain remaining 'trapped in literal present' with the 'stark and extreme possibility that, in the end, such people may have simply no identity'.

Observations in her book seem to be corroborated in a recent article, 'The neural basis of video gaming', appearing in the journal *Translational Psychiatry*.[278] While, according to research, 'video game playing can enhance visual skills related to attention and probabilistic inferences [as well as] improvements in higher cognitive executive functions', adverse effects have also been reported in the literature.[279,280]

In the study underpinning the *Translational Psychiatry* article, scientists found that '[t]eenagers who spend many hours playing video games developed brains similar to those of gamblers' and that 'video gaming is related to addiction'.[278] The researchers studied 154 healthy 14-year-olds, who played video games for an average of 12 hours a week, and scanned their brains while they played two games. The study demonstrated that 'those teenagers who spent more time play-ing on their computer had more grey matter in a part of the brain which is rich in dopamine, a chemical that makes us feel pleasure and reward'. While the scientists conclude that their 'results have implications for the understanding of the structural and functional basis of excessive but non-pathological video game playing', they do not allude to the psychological factors that may impact on teenagers' brains.

Scientists interviewed further to the study debate whether video gaming is related to addiction and see the value of the research in terms of 'giving us a better understanding of possible long-term treatment'.[278] Although these are praisewor-thy considerations, is there not a bigger question to be answered? That is, what can society do to ensure that video gaming – along with other computer-related gadgetry – does not get out of hand? As with other mental disorders or addictions, the consequences of spending too many hours playing video games – or social networking for that matter – can only be damaging to individual health, physical and mental, and to society as a whole.

There is a strong case to be made to those who profit from their inventions – while potentially doing harm to those who are most vulnerable in society – to assume collective moral and social responsibility for their actions. Not doing so may result in Professor Greenfield's scenario of the future being realised:

> Remember we are all looking back on the journey with minds shaped by the previous century, but we may soon lose the luxury of cynicism and compla-cency that may have engendered. If you are mobilised in the world of 'dreams and shadows', if you are free of pain yet mentally standardised, if you are living principally in a cyber-world or a chemical oblivion, then it may be only of secondary importance whether the rich countries alone undergo this trans-formation, or the developing world too. And it would no longer matter whether you, or they, had minds of their own. Time could be running out on the luxury of considering any options at all – who knows, we may be the last generation of individuals able, or willing, to have them.[4]

Still, today, far removed from this sad twenty-first-century prospect is the world of the poor. In a recent paper, *Educating a new generation of doctors to improve the health of populations in low-and middle income countries*,[281] the authors express the critical need 'to increase the number of doctors in low- and middle-income countries'. Making their case, and citing one example, they mention that '[w]hile sub-Saharan Africa has 24% of the global disease burden, it has only 3% of the world's health workers'. Although the number of doctors is clearly a key issue, there are also concerns, as indicated in *The Lancet* Commission report,[56] with 'the quality and relevancy of the providers of the future' necessitating 'a trans-formative approach to medical education'. According to the authors, fundamental changes are required that are 'defined by a commitment to social responsibility', and insist 'on inter-sectorial engagement to determine how students are recruited, educated, and deployed as doctors'. A systemic problem with existing medical education is that many 'educational institutions are isolated from national health systems and from health service delivery, limiting their ability to prepare graduates to respond to the evolving policies, epidemiology, and technologies relevant to their eventual practice sites'. The issues include a mismatch between university curricula and 'the disease burden of the areas in which doctors are most urgently needed', and '[t]raining physicians in isolation', thereby preparing them 'poorly for team-based practice'.

Global responses to the present situation include 'multi-sectorial innovation during the scale-up of medical education – ranging from new recruitment strategies, faculty development, and curriculum reform on the institutional level, to cross-sector planning and investment on the national level'. Further, the authors observe that matching evolving epidemiology, patient demographics, and health systems is particularly pressing in low- and middle-income countries, and that curricula need to incorporate 'community medicine and public health', making these 'compulsory rotations', and 'with a focus on prevention and determinants of health'. Moreover, the authors report that there is evidence that 'the most effective means of care delivery' occurs when tasks are partially transferred to non-physician providers. While an outstanding issue relates to recruiting the right students (e.g. from underserved areas), there is also a need 'for faculty with appropriate skills and experience to teach a new generation of providers' and to develop appropriate incentive structures.

Taking a wider view, the authors conclude, '[s]caling up medical education' – 'matching education to population needs – has implications for strategic planning and financial investment on a long-term and multi-sectorial basis'.

An attempt to ensure that patient needs are met was recently reported in a national study by the UK NHS Confederation entitled *Feeling Better? Improving the patient experience in hospital.*[282] The report was based on available data and the scrutiny of exemplary practice at seven leading hospitals (two in the United Kingdom, five in the United States). Emerging from comparative data were several interesting and directly applicable findings regarding common factors across successful health organisations:

- *Transformational leadership* – 'often a senior figure with a clear vision and drive'.
- Change is effected across the *whole system*, rather than in one corner.
- *Patients and their families are engaged* in care and those experiences are viewed from the users' perspectives.
- There is an emphasis on *continual feedback* from patients, families and carers and measurement for improvement.
- There is a consistent *integrated programme* of activities, rather than a series of small random projects.
- There is recognition of the importance of *embedding desired values and behaviours* across the organisation (this goes beyond lip service to a mission statement).
- *Staff are enabled* to deliver excellent patient experience and empowered to make changes themselves.
- There is greater *clinical engagement* and professional empowerment.

These factors may have implications for recruitment of senior staff and strategic planning, including systemic or holistic thinking and the importance of building values that are patient-based. One important factor that seems to be in place in leading hospitals is trust and empowerment and ongoing efforts to improve, a conclusion also reached in the Bennets's research[239] into identifying factors that underpin long-term and highly successful organisations. Trust, empowerment and the motivation to continually improve go hand in hand in successful change efforts. As Philip Collins, columnist and leader writer for *The Times*, rightly concludes '[g]ranting power to individuals improves service.' According to Collins '[l]eft-wing politicians once knew this.' Citing Michael Foot [former leader of the Labour party], who was 'talking about his hero, Aneurin Bevan' [architect of the NHS], Collins emphasises Bevan 'desperately wanted the patient to have free choice of doctor. He saw it as the best safeguard against poor service from the general practitioner.'[276]

People who are overly micromanaged – possibly a concern with a 'target culture' – tend to feel frustration and sometimes resentment, as most professionals are motivated in environments where they are able to think creatively (a natural human response to complex challenges) but responsibly. While this observation may be true in most cases, it does not apply to all, which may be a reason for the 'top-down' culture in some environments. For example, the NHS Confederation report highlights that at the interpersonal patient–doctor level there appears room for improvement with compassion being at the forefront of relationships and treatment. That there are serious difficulties in UK 'patient-centred care' (receiving a 7 out of 7 score, where 1 is excellent) – along with Canada (a score of 5) and the Netherlands (a score of 6) – was confirmed in the 2010 Commonwealth Fund study,[54] discussed in Chapter 1.

Both the Bennets's[239] and the NHS Confederation[282] research on factors across successful organisations recognise the importance of desired values and behaviours that 'fit with their culture and their standards'. The difference between the two philosophical assumptions, however, is that the Bennets present an account of essentially conservative or static factors that have traditionally underpinned successful organisations, and the NHS Confederation findings look toward a future, where 'what's in the past' may indeed no longer be 'prologue'. While we need to acknowledge that 'initiating change may upset the equilibrium', pursuing and sustaining desirable new directions may permit 'the achievement of a new equilibrium', which carries with it at least the potential of 'a full realisation of the intended benefits'.[283]

Fundamental to the rethinking of medical practice and medical education in the twenty-first century must inevitably be a rebalancing of the 'biological and body-focused'[284] medical model of practice, as mentioned earlier. The biomedical approach, which evolved during the twentieth century, largely as a result of scientific breakthroughs, increasingly needs to value the importance of cognitive, emotional, behavioural and social factors.[285,286] It may be worth recalling that, given the demographic changes occurring in British society, recommendations in a recent groundbreaking report on restructuring undergraduate medical education by the UK Royal College of General Practitioners and the Health Foundation clearly subscribe to a major reorientation in medical education.[211]

Distinguishing between two differing models and philosophical assumptions, Dr Mark Dombeck, former director of the US Mental Help Net, observes that 'medicine takes a mechanistic approach to illness'.[284] In other words, 'the physician tends to view patients in a detached way, as a body with a problem, much like an actual mechanic might try to figure out what was wrong with a car. … The physician determines a diagnosis based on her analysis of symptoms. Her prescription is designed to fix the diagnosed problem.' However, '[n]owhere in this chain of events is the physician encouraged to be particularly interested in the experience of the person behind the problem'. Further, Dr Dombeck notes that '[w]here the medical model tends to rely on cures that are external to the patient (like medicine), the psychological model tries to cure by getting the patient to use internal resources they already possess in a different way'.

Likely more feasible in community-based care, the goal of the physician–patient consultation changes,[200,211] as it will be largely based on 'forming a relationship with the patient and in using this relationship to help along the process of change' with a view 'to actively involve and motivate their patients to make the specified changes that will improve the patients' functioning. Reflecting the transference from industrial- to information-age care',[73] '[g]ood patients become active partners in the process of change'.[281] Both models have strengths and weaknesses', according to Dr Dombeck. 'Where medicine excels at crisis management and biological manipulation, psychology excels at behaviour change and growth.' While there are 'incompatibilities', he asserts, 'these two models need each other desperately, as [w]ithout the other model present as a balancing force, any one of these models would ignore vital facets of the human condition.'[284] Increasingly, recognising the contributions of each of these fields – along with the other social sciences – will have significant implications for the education and training of the healthcare workers. One of the struggles within medical schools – perhaps in other healthcare professions as well – continues to be the equal valuing of the arts and the humanities alongside the natural sciences and clinical medicine. Gautama Buddha (c. 563–483 BCE), a spiritual teacher from the Indian subcontinent and on whose teachings Buddhism was founded, may appropriately remind us that 'our sorrows and wounds are healed only when we touch them with compassion'.[286]

The bottom line of this book is that while national reports have called for vast improvements in medical education, international reports have gone further, seeking radical transformation of how all healthcare professionals in both developing and developed countries are educated and trained. Major drivers of change, as outlined previously, include the difficulty of recruiting sufficient healthcare workers in remote and rural areas; the imbalance between disease burden and available healthcare support; the mismatch between the healthcare curricula on offer and what is actually needed by patients; and the lack of opportunity for inter/trans-professional learning.

These challenges, according to the *Policy Forum* report authors, demand the development of 'a new generation of doctors who are better equipped to meet the evolving health needs of the communities they serve'.[281] In their view, and reflecting key reforms in *The Lancet* Commission report,[56] at all levels (international, national, local), the 'vision for transformative education' calls for the following.

- Greater alignment between educational institutions and the systems that are responsible for health service delivery.
- Country ownership of priorities and programming related to medical education, with political commitment and partnerships to facilitate reform at national, regional and local levels.
- Promotion of social accountability in medical education and of close collaboration with communities.
- Doctors who are clinically competent and provide the highest quality of care.
- Global excellence coupled with local relevance in medical research and education.
- Vibrant and sustainable medical education institutions with dynamic curricula and supportive learning environments, including good physical infrastructure.
- Faculty of outstanding quality who are motivated and can be retained.

Reflecting on both 'poor and rich countries' *The Lancet* commissioners advocate local problem-solving 'while harnessing the benefits of transnational flows of knowledge.'[56] Rising beyond national self-interests, they remind us that 'we increasingly' need to be mindful that we 'have one global [limited?] pool of health professional talent' and that primary health care needs to be accessible across the globe 'in very different contexts.' Recognising 'our growing interdependence in all health matters,' the commissioners also acknowledge two key developments that may foster greater transnational sharing in support of patient care: 'the movement abroad of schools in developed countries' which 'establish affiliated campuses in emerging economies,' and the fact that 'global health as a field is expanding rapidly in professional education' with '[c]entres, institutes, units and programs in global health'.

As another sign of global interdependence, albeit in financial matters – that of course have significant impact on healthcare providers and professionals – Dr Gerard Lyons, chief economist at Standard Chartered Bank, comments in an informative article, 'How emerging economies help global growth',[287] that we 'might find it hard to believe', but worldwide 'the world economy has grown by 14% and is set to reach US$52 trillion by the end of this year' compared with a decade ago when 'it was only US$24 trillion'. Most of this considerable growth is attributable to the emerging world led by China, including Latin America, where there is continued strong demand for commodities from China, as well as from robust credit growth.

Reminiscent of economist Roger Bootle's[2] arguments in the Introduction, Dr Lyons also provides several reasons why emerging economies will help global growth. First, unlike the West and in contrast to the fundamentals in Europe, where there has been 'an overhang of debt ... and the confidence has been shot to pieces', in the emerging world 'the policy cupboard is almost full and confidence is likely to prove resilient' with China – projected to overtake the US economy by 2027[288] – becoming the 'largest export market for Japan, Korea, South-East Asia and Australia, the second largest for the EU [European Union], Brazil and South Africa, and even the third largest for Germany, Canada, the US and the UK'. Second, China is able to 'support growth at home and across the globe'. Third, 'domestic demand is relatively solid across large parts of Africa and Asia', reflecting 'investment, infrastructure, spending, employment growth and economic diversification'. While many threats remain for UK small and medium-sized businesses, Dr Lyons advises that there are also many opportunities 'to become more global in their outlook',[287] including, of course, employment possibilities for healthcare professionals.

International beacons of change and innovation in medical education

In the Western world, we have come a long and often circuitous way since medicine and medical education began to make a difference in people's lives; some would say from the days of the 'wise woman' in the seventeenth and eighteenth centuries or before, or the 1880s; others, from the 1930s with the development of the first antibiotic to fight infectious diseases. Life expectancy has almost doubled in the past 100 years but, despairingly, not in most developing nations, where huge inequalities and inequities in health and social care remain, and where in some geographical locations (e.g. Somalia) things are actually deteriorating.

Today there are many institutional and organisational examples in developed and developing countries where innovative medical education thinking has been turned into practical reality. These and other developments in high-income countries, 'where standard models of health and health systems are based around physicians, hospitals, technology and an exclusive professionalism' need to be 'spread across the globe', as advocated by Lord Crisp[258] and *The Lancet* commissioners generally.[56]

In Canada, McMaster's pioneering medical school's problem-based learning initiative in the late 1960s and early 1970s definitely places the School at the forefront of innovation in medical education.[289] As it subscribes to constructivist (personal meaning-making through social interaction) and situated learning principles (learning in a 'community of practice'), the educational concept is one the very few truly transformational innovations in higher education generally that has philosophically, structurally and processually been changing the face of medical education across the globe.

The Melbourne School of Medicine in Australia has initiated the only Australian professional-entry masters level programme, the Melbourne MD [Doctor of Medicine]. Planners believe that the new programme 'creates a new benchmark in 21st century medical education'.[290] The programme is based on meeting key competencies and attributes in six domains (Self, Knowledge, Patient, Medical Profession, Systems of Health Care and Society). Key features include an annual interdisciplinary student-led component and an integrative transition final-year capstone component.

In the United States the University of Michigan Medical School, 'one of the top two or three public medical schools in the nation', with its many firsts, including the first woman graduate in 1871, collaboration across disciplines, and with its present wider focus through Global Reach – 'to make the world a better place' – is definitely another.[291] The Harvard Initiative for Global Health, including the recent partnership initiative between Massachusetts General Hospital and Harvard Medical School in the development of a new internal medicine residency programme in global primary care, represents another groundbreaking innovation.[115] With its transformative medical innovations, starting in 1889, Johns Hopkins Medicine continues to stand out, as one example, with its Internet Learning Center, 'now in use at one out of every three internal medicine residency training programs' in the United States.[292]

A 'beacon of change and innovation' in the UK is the University of Southampton's Faculty of Medicine, having celebrated 40 years (1971–2011) of medicine with over 5000 graduates at the University.[293] The Faculty, under the leadership of Professor Iain Cameron, dean, and Dr Christopher Stephens, University and faculty director of education, responding to the GMC's various updates of *Tomorrow's Doctors*, initiated a number of reforms (e.g. early patient contact, a systems-based curriculum approach, a study in depth in the students' penultimate year), along with a strong emphasis on staff and educational development generally at both undergraduate and postgraduate levels. In addition, the Faculty is committed to fostering the role of research in medicine (in particular in such areas as climate change, the ageing population, high-tech crime and lifestyle diseases). The Staff

Development function, under the direction of Dr Faith Hill, has been recognised as a model for supporting clinicians in terms of teaching and learning across the UK.

Moreover, the highly regarded BM6 programme, which started in 2002, and whose main focus, under the guidance of Carolyn Blundell, has been a six year 'Widening Access to Medicine' programme to meet both the national agenda of widening participation to medicine from more diverse backgrounds. An innovative BM4 graduate entry programme, spearheaded by Dr Jenny Field, commenced in 2004 and is one of the few that is open to graduates with *any* degree. Similarly, the School's curriculum and quality initiatives, including the incorporation of key vertical themes (communications, law and ethics, diversity, and novel 'interprofessional' learning programme, working with 11 other health and social care disciplines across two universities), have been identified as bringing a present and future orientation to the Bachelor of Medicine (BM) curricula.

Paralleling the University's innovative mission and aims, the focus on the 'student learning experience' has been paramount in all of the Faculty's decision-making and policy developments. Its new partnership with health provider, Gesundheit Nordhessen Holding, based in Kassel, will also allow German students to be taught in Southampton before returning to Germany for the latter part of their education, and is consistent with *The Lancet* Commission recommendations to expand healthcare student/trainee opportunities globally. The beneficiaries of these innovations are decidedly the medical students – and likely all other health/social care students – preparing for a career in health or social care and, most importantly, future patients or clients.

In terms of postgraduate training, the United Kingdom Kent, Surrey & Sussex (KSS) Postgraduate Deanery's guiding philosophy underpinning education, curriculum, trainee and supervisor support, as well as its quality management systems, merit special attention.[294] All of the Deanery work 'is informed by a Principled Approach to Practice with its starting point taking 'an explicitly ethical stance, summarised as Kant's Categorical Imperative: "treat others as you wish to be treated yourself"'.[295] And, '[w]ith those principles foregrounded,' the Deanery moves 'directly into the real-life, complex, problematic world of everyday clinical practice' with the 'intention to develop practical solutions to practical problems, drawing on a wide range of theoretical perspectives.' The Deanery's approach to quality management is therefore 'highly collaborative', 'developmental', for both trusts and the Deanery, and 'flexible', encouraging 'local diversity and creativity within regional and national guidelines'. At the core of the Deanery's 'collaborative practice' is the 'professional conversation', which is 'an ongoing discussion with stakeholders about principles, processes and patients'. The Deanery's Quality Management System (QMS) contains five key elements: Contract Review; a wide range of Academic Development programmes for supervisors, teachers, trainees, administrators; GEAR (Graduate Education and Assessment Regulations);

KSS School (Specialty) Development; and Medical Workforce Management. Considered collectively, Deanery initiatives represent worthy examples of 'creativity, innovation, and continuous improvement' along with efforts at 'supporting excellence through effective policy'.[102]

Reflecting on health systems in the Far East, there can be no doubt that China's Peking University Medical School (PUMC) well deserves to be among global leaders in medical education.[296] In an exchange of correspondence between Professor Yuan-Fang Chen, vice chair of the Expert Committee for Education at PUMC, and Dr Chen, president of the China Medical Board (CMB), and co-chair of *The Lancet* Commission,[56] she highlights the contributions PUMC has made 'to deserve the honour as "the cradle of modern medicine in China."' Observing that PUMC 'set a norm for medical and pre-medical education and residency training' in China in the 1920s and 1930s, she ascribes the success of PUMC to following Flexnerian ideals[121,125] – particularly the mantra 'no science, no medical truth' and emphasising the importance of 'real life teaching' (learning process), as well as recognising the hidden curriculum – especially 'the role modeling of humanistic care'.

As stated by Professor Chen, two key directions need to continue to inform medical education: 'global health in medical science' and the 'promotion of public health', and, consistent with Flexner's philosophy, 'formal analytic thinking and the integration of basic science, research and clinical teaching'. And, while identifying serious pitfalls in China's medical education system – in particular the proliferation of 8-year medical schools and placing quantity over quality, she acknowledges that there is need for 'instillation of new philosophy, new tenets and new operating systems to bring about radical change, rather than just making some superficial improvements'. In responding to Professor Yuan-Fang Chen, and noting that there is 'more agreement than differences' in their views, President Chen of the CMB, while agreeing in large measure with her views, reinforces the need for enhancing interprofessional teamwork and expanding the diversity of medical professionals along with the 'integration of community-based and humanistic learning in a natural science-dominated curriculum'.

In this thoughtful exchange, there appears to be common ground not only that 'Flexner's legacy will be ever-lasting and universal' but also for the need 'to examine where changing contexts are compelling changing responses'. In China – and possibly in other countries – transformations are urgently needed that 'go beyond surface achievements', the 'chase for winning honours' and the necessity of prioritising quality of care over quantity measures. At its deepest roots, medicine and medical education must continue to be about meeting the health needs of all citizens in each community.

Perhaps the two exemplary interventions that illustrate success of community-based care and which hold the potential of making a real difference in many developing countries reside in the Philippines. The first relates to developments at the Ateneo de Zamboanga University School of Medicine. Here the faculty was successful in dramatically reducing the infant mortality rate – made possible by 'a spirit of volunteerism' and 'the social accountability model of preferential local student selection'.[229] To counter the 'brain drain' that is occurring in the Philippines, and the 'maldistribution of health manpower prevailing in the country in the 1970s', planners developed an innovative 5-year healthcare curriculum to prepare students to serve in underserved areas. Students enter a stepladder curriculum that begins with community-health worker training and practice (midwifery), then a BA in Nursing and for some a BSc in Community Health. Finally, students may qualify to enter the MD programme, which 'alternates didactics, community work and clinical work. Graduates then complete National Physicians Licensure Exams.' Only about 10% of those trained have gone abroad,[153] compared with the 50%–100% migration rate of various graduating classes of the University of the Philippines College of Medicine over the years. The important point is that based on follow-up of graduates, the majority practise in underserved rural areas rather than in the big cities or abroad. As a sign that the model achieves key human resource aims, it has now also been adopted in two other provinces, Quezon province (the new school is located in Baler) and South Cotabato (in Koronadal City).

The final 'beacon of change and innovation' – although there are many more internationally, nationally and locally that could be cited across the globe than space allows in this book – recognises the work of The Secretariat and The Advisory Committee engaged in the Sub-Saharan African Medical Schools Study (SAMSS).[297] The SAMSS was funded by the Bill and Melinda Gates Foundation and housed within the George Washington University, DC, School of Public Health Services, with Fitzhugh Mullan MD as Principal Investigator and Seble Frehywopt MD MSHA, co-chair of the SAMSS Advisory Committee.

To gain a realistic perspective on the world health situation, it is crucial to note that 'Africa suffers 24% of the world's total burden of disease but has only 3% of the world's health workforce, including 1.5% of the world's physician workforce.' And, as mentioned in Chapter 1, the physician to population ratio is alarming with 'an estimated ratio of 18/100 000, as compared to other countries, such as India (60/100 000), Brazil (170/100 000), and the United States (270/100 000).' The problems are compounded as there are only 169 medical schools in the 48 countries with many of the 10 000 physicians per year leaving to work in other countries. The SAMSS study, 'landscaping in nature' and with site visits to 10 medical schools between May 2009 and February 2010, sought 'to help provide a platform of understanding regarding the status, trends and present and future capacity building efforts for educators, policy makers, and international organisations.'

Innovations and recommendations that were identified in the SAMSS included 'educational planning that focuses on national health needs'; 'international partnerships'; 'curricula innovations', such as fostering 'critical thinking and community-based education(CBE)', 'the teaching of family medicine and 'public health and plans for the use of telehealth and distance learning'; recognising the role of 'private medical schools'; and the need for 'establishing national and regional post-graduate medical education programmes.'

The recommendations that flow from the issues and innovations identified reinforce the view that '[s]trong health systems are central to the attainment of health equity' and that 'lack of human resources is a key obstacle to the attainment of strong health systems.' There is no question that '[p]hysicians are a core component of the human resource pool, and that Sub-Saharan Africa needs more physicians while ensuring the quality and relevance of medical school graduates.' Further, '[i]t also needs strong medical schools … which are accredited to assure quality, well resourced, and relevant to national health needs.' With population increases in the next 30–40 years in many nations increasing by over 300%, it is crucial that the issues and recommendation from the SAMSS are not only taken forward but also that they achieve the ends that The Secretariat and The Advisory Committee envisaged. Failing to do so would be a recipe for disaster rather than an opportunity for re-balancing global health on this planet or ensuring the well-being of its people.

Medical and healthcare education at a crossroad

The possibility exists that medical education could play a more vital role in helping to shape the future of healthcare. Its most powerful contribution – working collaboratively with other health professionals – may be to provide opportunities for debating basic social, instructional and institutional issues relating to the future of populations and healthcare, and to help shape new educational frameworks and approaches in order to 'match professional education and the realities of health service delivery'.[56] The proposed reforms at national and international levels outlined in this book perhaps present a unique opportunity for decision-makers to engage in much needed transformation of healthcare – rather than, as Roy Porter, concluded several years ago, 'merely a ragbag of cost-capping initiatives, accounting and managerial strategies and short-term economics' that seem to characterise improvements in medical systems in the last few decades.[232]

Addressing these serious problems in practical terms will not be easy, as affirmed by Samuel Thier, professor emeritus of Medicine and Health Care Policy at Harvard University. Speaking at the launch of *The Lancet* Commission report,[56] Professor Thier reminds us that transforming 'the education of the professions is a daunting task', but that '[h]aving that education informed by and responsible to the needs of health systems is an even more daunting task'.[147] While confirming that the issues were clear along with the imaginative solutions, he wisely cautioned that the larger vision needed to be brought down to 'a practical human scale in size and location'.

Although the teaching of medicine 'is inescapably embedded in the social environment',[221] common aspirations of the 'vision for transformative education', discussed earlier – that crosses the developed and developing educational worlds – will be for planners at all levels to find meaningful ways of building 'an insistence on excellence'[102] into the professional formation of physicians and other healthcare professions.

'Taking responsibility for excellence' in patient care would mean that learners, practitioners and policymakers would be 'incorporated into microsystems dedicated to improvement in quality'. This refocusing would increase the probability of achieving 'the best outcomes for a patient or patients collectively',[102] regardless of geographical, environmental or social context.

Echoing the eight criteria set by the Picker Institute Europe for evaluating healthcare services,[209] the UK Social Care Institute for Excellence[298] concludes that, according to evidence-based research, good healthcare depends on eight 'dignity factors' – all of which ideally 'need to be present in care'. While implementing these 'factors' would require considerable investment of resources, particularly in the developing world, where most of these factors are far removed from present realities, even possibilities, they are crucial gold standards in quality care for all nations. In terms of all healthcare providers, they demand a 'new professionalism'[56] 'that supports and promotes a person's self-respect', or, essentially the best care that professionals have to offer.

1. *Choice and control*: enabling people to make choices about the way they live and the care they receive.
2. *Communication*: speaking to people respectfully and listening to what they have to say.
3. *Eating and nutritional care*: providing a choice of nutritious, appetising meals that meet the needs and choices of individuals and support with eating where needed.
4. *Pain management*: ensuring that people living with pain have the right help and medication to reduce suffering and improve their quality of life.
5. *Personal hygiene*: enabling people to maintain their usual standards of personal hygiene.
6. *Practical assistance*: enabling people to maintain their independence but providing 'that little bit of help'.
7. *Privacy*: respecting people's personal space, privacy in personal care and confidentiality of personal communication.

8. *Social inclusion*: supporting people to keep in contact with family and friends, and to participate in social activities.

Professor Steve Field, who led the recent NHS Futures Forum in Britain,[299] probably had these ends in mind when he concluded that the transformation that is necessary in healthcare can only be achieved 'if strong leaders at all levels, whether from a clinical or managerial backgrounds, articulate a clear vision, embrace innovation, promote collaboration and champion change'.

Further, he advises, '[t]he system must support them to do this by aligning levers and incentives and facilitating the sharing of best practice'. And, giving sage advice that may be relevant for all health systems undergoing change, he stresses the importance of learning 'the lessons of implementation' and evaluating 'the individual and combined impact of the reforms' and adapting 'solutions in the interests of driving even better outcomes for patients'.[299]

Similar resolve for change is now increasingly heard globally. As another example, in an annual address to members of the Institute of Medicine, President Fineberg advanced a number of fundamental reforms that would radically improve healthcare in the United States.[300] On top of his list, which includes research support, costs, comparative effectiveness research, health information technologies, physician payment and medical education, as well as informed patient preferences, to name several areas for reform, is *prevention of disease*.

Prevention, he argues, usually 'gets short shrift as when it works it is invisible; it typically takes a long time for benefits to be realised; and it often demands daily, consistent changes in lifestyle and ingrained habits that are hard to maintain' but 'can have high payoffs'. In his concluding remarks, he cautions his audience to 'not neglect the nation's public health infrastructure; promotion of nutritious and healthful diets, healthy and safe environments; healthy families and healthy communities and preparedness to detect and respond to natural and human-initiated threats to health'.

Research findings, practitioner and family stories are, therefore, reliably evidencing that the best patient outcomes are shaped by a combination of appropriate and timely medical interventions, along with kindness, compassion and empathy. While these are essential cornerstones of any sound relationship, we must also recognise that in many developing or poor countries people can only 'dream' of doctors, nurses, medication, good health and leading long, healthy, productive lives. By most measures, it seems that the West still has much to be thankful for despite the prevailing and uncertain forces of change.

However, unless we learn lessons from the past we remain vulnerable. In an introspective and anonymous piece, appearing in a collection of short essays on global sustainability,[301] the anonymous writer notes that the 'residents of the ancient metropolis of Ephesus (the best preserved classical city of the Eastern Mediterranean) never considered the impermanence of their home'. After all, 'they were part of the Roman Empire, the most powerful empire on earth, one of the most desirable cities in the civilised world, with a population of at least 250,000.' Today,

> Ephesus is an amazing testament to the engineering and of its Greek and Roman former residents. And yet, for the past 1,500 years, after river silt destroyed its harbour, Ephesus has remained a dead city. The lessons of the Ephesians are very practical. Two thousand years ago, its residents assumed that Ephesus would be teeming with children, merchants and politicians as long as there was a sunrise.

Of course, that was not to be and, unlike the Ephesians, the writer cautions, '[w]e can't assume, that we can continue to do things as we've always done and still go on forever'.

The most important lesson from the Ephesians – and possibly our most fervent challenge in this century – may be not allowing 'things to happen because of our reluctance to alter course'. The other – perhaps even more daunting aspiration – as William Joy philosophically pointed out in the Introduction to this book, is understanding 'what we can and should relinquish in this century' and 'finding consensus on where society wants or needs to go' in order to 'make our future much less dangerous'.[8]

Viewed from a historical perspective, achieving these ends seems beyond reach at this point. However, moving towards sustainability – better management of the ecosystem and consumption of resources, and, in particular, acknowledging that conflicts between and across nations, based most often delusionally on self-interest and resource 'control', rather than on resource 'sharing' to benefit those most in need, we have few options. And, as highlighted in Chapter 1, we urgently have to stop 'doing a lot of things to save us from ourselves'.[301] Moreover, while medicine has advanced tremendously in the last sixty years or so, especially, according to Dr James Le Fanu, between the post-war period to the late 1970s, one of his main conclusions in *The Rise and Fall of Modern Medicine* is that 'the virtues of imagination and perseverance' of modern medicine have all too often given 'way to the vices of hubris and self-deception'.[302]

Moreover, while he recognises that 'medicine will continue to be a powerful and immensely successful enterprise, ameliorating the chronic diseases associated with ageing and, where possible saving the lives of the actual ill', discontents will likely remain within the medical profession itself and with the public. The former, he suggests, because of possible 'regrets' of their chosen career, and the public, because they have become 'neurotically concerned about their health', largely spurred on by the pharmaceutical industry and 'its obsession with the new', and 'the prospect of windfall profits while they remain under patent'. These profits, Le Fanu argues, are 'the lifeblood that drives the industry forward', taking 'the form of "better but more expensive mousetraps" or indeed "useless mouse-traps," promoted on the grounds that they are better than no mousetraps at all'. In his concluding comments Dr Le Fanu reaffirms that '[g]enuine progress, optimistic and forward-looking, is always to be welcomed, but progress as an ideological necessity leads to obscurantism, falsehood and corruption'.

Perhaps now really is the time, according to James Le Fanu – also affirmed by both WHO director-general Margaret Chan in Chapter 1 and Jerome Groopman, professor of medicine at Harvard, in Chapter 7 – 'to relocate medicine back within that tradition so eloquently evoked by Sir William Osler'.[120] Le Fanus's central argument seems to be that '[i]f the practical limits of what medicine can legitimately achieve' were understood and recognised, then '[t]he timeless virtues of judgement and good sense might then triumph over the shallow restlessness of the present through a reaffirmation of the personal relationship between doctor and patient' [302,303]

It should be clear that neither the developed nor the developing world can afford to continue as they are. While each of these 'worlds' has unique challenges, and there are of course many socio-economic and political variations within these nations, there is a pressing need to accelerate bridging or exchange of ideas, and to share the wealth, including knowledge capital, of the relatively few (in numbers) with the poverty of the many. Unquestionably, our survival as a species – environmental, economic and social – in the twenty-first century depends on viable transformative change in each of these arenas (and, crucially, in *us*). The late Roy Porter, eminent medical historian and Professor Emeritus at the Centre for the History of Medicine (University College London [UCL]), postulated over a decade ago that 'investment in public health, environmental hygiene and better nutrition would do far more' for the developing world, than 'sophisticated clinical medicine programmes'.[232]

At the level of the individual patient – for whom this book is really all about – we must insist that care is provided by healthcare professionals who are able to consistently demonstrate competence, integrity, teamwork, caring and compassion,[304,305] – especially for the most vulnerable in society.[306] These capacities can be optimised by:

- creating health and social care programmes that meet population needs through much improved workforce strategic planning at regional, national, and international levels[307–309]
- ensuring that the quality and safety of patient care are the primary focus of all training programmes[310]
- incorporating within healthcare curricula inter/trans-professional learning

approaches that nurture the self-worth, mutual respect and dignity of patients and colleagues

- finding the right balance between curative and preventive care in healthcare curricula
- personalising the learning experience of students and trainees to allow learning to be centred around individual needs and consider the learners' preferred style, approaches and pace of learning
- increasing opportunities to share and access high-quality global resources that are learner-centred and suitable for twenty-first century healthcare professionals through use of the information technologies[56]
- providing occasions for system-wide placements or clerkships, nationally and internationally, particularly considering the health burdens of poor countries.

A closing word and the 'pale blue dot'

Finally, in many ways this book is about re-balancing the health inequities that exist across the planet, particularly between rich and poor countries. One of the most crucial examples relates to the worldwide shortage of c. 4.5 million healthworkers, causing a crisis in at least 57 countries, as evidenced in annual World Health Organization reports.[11,13,61,281] With patient to doctor ratios ranging from c. 400:1 in developed nations to as high as c. 50,000:1 in sub-Saharan Africa, which has 24% of the world's disease burden, but only 3% of the world's healthworkers, and just 1.5% of the world's physician workforce, the message cannot be more stark or disheartening.

Other disturbing lifestyle patterns are also highlighted in the book. The alarming rise of obesity in most nations with associated health problems – cancers, heart disease, diabetes – could in due course bankrupt health systems. These trends are taking place while the number of people living in extreme poverty and who are malnourished – in both developing and developed nations – has ballooned to over 1.6 billion (more than one out of seven of the world's population!).

The book also raises concerns about the unsustainable costs of healthcare, with many countries facing insurmountable debts, while, at the same time, there is the growing need to ensure that the elderly are cared for with respect, compassion and dignity. It also points out that 'medicating for life', including prescribing antipsychotic drugs to children as young as five (along with rampant drug usage across all ages), is on the rise worldwide and is 'a slow fuse to disaster'.

Moreover, while health professions work together to care for patients, the book questions why these students and trainees, continue, in the main, to develop their knowledge and skills separately. Richard Horton, editor-in-chief of *The Lancet*, in his commentary on *The Lancet* Commission report, observes that lack of progress in building 'a new kind of professionalism – patient-centred, interprofessional, and team-based' can be traced to 'the rigid and damaging tribalism that afflicts the professions today'. Further, he asserts 'what the Commission argues for is nothing less than a remoralisation of health professionals' education'.[311] Echoing the Commission report,[56] the book advocates consideration of new curriculum models that are more inclusive, integrative and that match health needs to competencies and training required for 21st century patients.

Conclusions reached by two Canadian medical practitioners, Professor Alex Jadad, founder and Chief Innovator of the Centre for Global eHealth Innovation at the University of Toronto, and Murray Enkin, Emeritus Professor of Obstetrics and Gynaecology at McMaster University, may be particularly germane to the book's themes. In their view 'computer technology can help us achieve optimal levels of health and well-being regardless of who or where we are – by transcending our cognitive, physical, institutional, geographical, cultural, linguistic, and historical boundaries'.[259] Or, as Baroness Susan Greenfield, a neuroscientist, also deduced in her recent book,[277] computer technology 'can contribute to our extinction ... the choice is ours' [259]

Taking their points forward, our future will undoubtedly depend on the collective wisdom and political will of informed planners making the right choices throughout the 21st century. In particular, these leaders will need to learn how best to manage change and transitions that have as their primary goal the betterment of the human condition. One of their main challenges – at global, national and community levels – may be finding the right balance in terms of 'materialism', technology and fundamental human values – especially recognising the centrality of the family unit, its place in the community and its future.[312,313]

FIGURE 10.1 The 'pale blue dot': photograph taken from Voyager 1 (launched 1977) on 14 February 1990, from the outer edge of the solar system, approximately 4 billion miles away (and now approximately 11 billion miles away), showing the Earth as a pale blue dot in a sunbeam

Look again at that dot. That's here. That's home. That's us. On it every-one you love, everyone you know, everyone you ever heard of, every human being who ever was, lived out their lives. The aggregate of our joy and suffering, thousands of confident religions, ideologies, and economic doctrines, every hunter and forager, every hero and coward, every creator and destroyer of civilization, every king and peasant, every young couple in love, every mother and father, hopeful child, inventor and explorer, every teacher of morals, every corrupt politician, every 'superstar,' every 'supreme leader,' every saint and sinner in the history of our species lived there – on a mote of dust suspended in a sunbeam.

The Earth is a very small stage in a vast cosmic arena. Think of the riv-ers of blood spilled by all those generals and emperors, so that, in glory and triumph, they could become the momentary masters of a fraction of a dot. Think of the endless cruelties visited by the inhabitants of one corner of this pixel on the scarcely distinguishable inhabitants of some other corner, how frequent their misunderstandings, how eager they are to kill one another, how fervent their hatreds.

Our posturings, our imagined self-importance, the delusion that we have some privileged position in the Universe, are challenged by this point of pale light. Our planet is a lonely speck in the great enveloping cosmic dark. In our obscurity, in all this vastness, there is no hint that help will come from elsewhere to save us from ourselves.

—Professor Carl Sagan (1934–96)[314]

Epilogue

Leadership in medicine and healthcare for the 21st century

Ruth Collins-Nakai MD MBA FRCPC MACC, **Chair, Canadian Medical Foundation, Ottawa, ON, Canada**

Over the past several decades there has been a continuous flow of resources dedicated to both management and leadership. More recently, the focus has been on governance as one of the tools of leadership. This is true of the business, not-for-profit, government, academic and, yes, even the healthcare sectors. The future sustainability of healthcare systems is increasingly being attributed to 'under-management' or 'under-leadership' or both. Why the search for good leadership? Why do physicians still resist accepting senior leadership positions? What follows is one approach to demonstrate the symbiotic relationship between good leadership and good management.

First, there are many definitions of both management and leadership. Some suggest that management deals with daily operations or 'doing things right', whereas leadership deals with opportunities and challenges or 'doing the right things'. Leadership can be defined as 'the capacity to influence others to act toward a common constructive purpose'.[315,316] Each of the concepts embedded in this definition is important for they beg questions about how to make good systems better. Questions such as: 'how do we develop leadership capacity, both organisationally and personally?'

For purposes of this Epilogue, we will assume good management in the healthcare system – recognising that many would say this is a large assumption, given what they see as inefficiencies in the system. We take this stand to focus our attention squarely on the challenges of leadership ... doing the right things!

There can be no doubt that public healthcare systems throughout the world are in transition: all are attempting to deliver more quality services with limited

human and other resources and in a sustainable fashion for the future. And this, while populations are both growing and growing older, with all that implies in terms of increased severity of chronic diseases. Technology also continues to evolve but its effects in terms of impact on health are often difficult to assess.

The combined impact of demography and technology is clear, however. Governments worldwide are facing structural deficits and sovereign debt has become the preoccupation of world leaders. If publicly-funded health and social systems are to survive in developed countries, and if improved health is to be attained in developing countries, leaders will have to come together to formulate shared objectives, values, directions, goals and metrics for the systems.

In the past, it has been surmised that leaders are 'born' to lead, with searches in the business world for people with the right temperament or charisma. Increasingly, however, it is recognised that leadership capabilities can be acquired through appropriately designed, strength-based educational development programmes.

Physicians have often been seen and have seen themselves as the 'natural' leaders in their communities. But neither admission criteria for entry into medical school, nor many undergraduate and postgraduate training programmes, emphasise leadership potential or skills development. As healthcare became more organised into complex systems and less attached to communities, professional administrators (managers) were increasingly legislated into the systems. Understandably, few physicians were attracted to move out of their clinical comfort zone to take on these challenges.

With the realisation that healthcare leadership challenges have moved from relatively 'tame' or manageable to complex, interdependent 'wicked' problems with no easy or obvious solutions, we now need to understand the emerging discipline of leadership better and then apply this better understanding to the unique challenges facing today's leaders.

Numerous competency frameworks for physician leadership have been developed, ranging from the Royal College of Physicians and Surgeons of Canada's *CanMEDS Framework*, the Canadian Medical Association's Physician Management Institutes (which, despite the reference to Management, actually has been reframed to focus on systematic leadership development), to The Academy of Medical Royal Colleges and the NHS Institute for Innovation and Improvement's *Medical Leadership Competency Framework* in the UK.[97]

The focus of essentially all such frameworks is still largely weighted toward achieving efficiency improvements through improved teamwork and collaboration among healthcare providers and through enhanced communication both among team members and with patients. These traditional frameworks also tend to focus on achieving better (patient) outcomes and system performance. All tend to dictate prescriptive competencies to be attained and maintained over time. Such frameworks are based on the traditional approaches to learning by acquiring specific, often very complex, knowledge. Yet with clinical knowledge growing exponentially year over year, one cannot 'learn' and retain all pertinent knowledge. This is why there is a growing recognition, for example in the UK and with the Association of Faculties of Medical Schools report, that medical education must be seriously revamped.[101]

Through improved measurements and expanded clinical trials, we have also discovered that there is a huge gap between what we as clinicians *know* and what we *do*, which becomes especially important in medicine where new knowledge and guidelines should help to transform and improve the care of our patients. It is increasingly clear that our hierarchical, rules- and power-based, somewhat rigid health leadership and management mechanisms are failing: failing to focus adequately on our patients and their increasingly complex needs, failing to find solutions to the growing health gaps between rich and poor, failing to bridge the increasing gaps between different healthcare providers, failing to control healthcare spending, failing to recognise and incorporate the growing number of women in medicine, failing to refocus services on prevention and what is actually good for the population, and failing to continue medicine as a caring profession.

So, in short, today's leadership is failing to adequately reflect the political, economic, sociological, technological and, above all, cultural realities of today's healthcare systems.

The present book about educating healthcare professions for the 21st century discusses the needs of the population and the over-burdened curriculum and opens the door to include new educational frameworks on leadership development. Leadership by physicians can no longer be taken for granted or assumed but must be nurtured, in particular as the notion of 'shared leadership' and 'shared accountability' for effective and safe patient care has been taking hold. Underlying these developments is recognising the importance of self-regulated teamwork,[99] in both hospital and, increasingly, in community settings, where team members agree to ensure that team members co-operate in meeting the shared objective of providing optimal care for all patients, and to take appropriate action when the outcomes are not satisfactory. To these ends, it appears that much can also be learned by healthcare professionals from crew resource management (CRM), a team training model from the aviation field.[316]

Ideally, leadership development would start in infants and young children. As we increasingly understand the development of the brain and the disastrous effects adverse childhood events can have on brain development, and as we recognise the optimisation of resiliency that can develop with quality early child learning and care, we begin to recognise the need for truly life-long learning if we are to develop wise leaders in the future. And what, you say, does the development of resiliency in pre-school children have to do with leadership in medicine and healthcare?

One of the first and most important characteristics of modern leadership is the ability to be self-reflective: that is, able to assess one's own values, biases, principles, motivations and, indeed, weaknesses and be able to use that information to learn, grow and change. Adults have great difficulty doing this if they have not developed resilience and the ability to critique and improve self in childhood. Adults who are dealing, consciously or not, with the devils of their past are influenced by their need to fulfill self-interests and have difficulty responding maturely and rationally to emotionally charged situations. We can no longer afford to have leaders experiencing power struggles or promulgating strategies based on ego or self-interest.

Other characteristics of a new leadership perspective would include an evidence base, a reliable mechanism to include change management (which helps people adapt to new frameworks and perceptions), an approach to systems thinking and the introduction of life-long learning in leadership.

One of the newest health leadership capabilities frameworks which has just these characteristics is 'LEADS in a Caring Environment', created jointly by the Health Care Leadership Association of British Columbia, the Canadian College of Health Leaders and the Canadian Health Leadership Network (CHLNet). This framework envisions an 'enhanced understanding and culture of leadership across the Canadian health system'. It is focused on five descriptive capabilities (**L**ead self, **E**ngage others, **A**chieve results, **D**evelop coalitions and **S**ystem transformation).[317] LEADS represents the collective wisdom of the current literature on the emerging discipline of leadership and its adaptation to complex systems such as healthcare. Originally commissioned by the Centre for Health Leadership and Research at the Royal Roads University in Victoria, British Columbia, LEADS has now been adopted as a preferred leadership platform right across Canada. Because this framework is capabilities-based (a concept familiar to physicians and other healthcare professionals), the skills developed should result in a maturing of relationship capabilities, including collaborative problem solving.

Indeed, there are an increasing number of health programmes in Canada that are adopting the LEADS framework. These include many provincial government health departments, the Canadian Medical Association, the Canadian Society of Physician Executives, Accreditation Canada, many health provider organisations, various health service organisations and now an educational institution, the Ryerson College of Nursing.

That is not to say that other groups are not recognising the need for leadership development within their organisations. Britain's National Health Service (NHS) Future Forum Report on Clinical Advice and Leadership has also recommended multi-professional clinical leadership, continuing professional development and support for leadership activities across NHS organisations but the details of exactly what they want developed in their people are missing.[318]

Let us assume for a moment that we are able to develop strong leaders in healthcare. What would we expect would change in the various systems that are present today? What are the metrics for success?

Ideally, appropriate care would be provided respectfully to those who need it, when they need it and where they need it. All children would have the opportunity for quality learning and care. Social determinants of health would be addressed by coordinated government policies, based on evidence provided by medicine and science. As a result, we would see less poverty, which would then cascade into less criminality, less mental illness, higher educational attainment and lower rates of chronic illness, less resolution of conflict through violence and improved productivity. Most healthcare would be provided in the community with hospitals playing a lesser role for the average citizen. Leaders, in both society and healthcare, would be courageous enough to act in the best interests of the populations they serve rather than in the best interests of business or economics.

In such a utopian scenario, it is likely that population and public health, paediatric and geriatric health, preventive health and acute illnesses would be provided through government systems and that most chronic diseases, specialty services and preferential add-ons would be provided through some type of partnership between the public and private sectors. This scenario is obviously distanced from today's health systems but by providing leadership training throughout the healthcare system to diverse groups of providers, there is an opportunity for influencing both health and societal outcomes, and for putting healthcare on a sustainable trajectory serving the populations most burdened.

It is not possible to reform or transform our current healthcare systems without leadership development. We cannot become more efficient or effective without better leadership. Paraphrasing Jim Collins in *Good to Great and the Social Sectors*,[319] it is imperative 'to make sure the right decisions happen – no matter how difficult or painful – for the long-term greatness of the institution and the achievement of its mission, independent of consensus or popularity'.[318] This is the challenge we face in healthcare: ensuring that appropriate decisions are made now for the long-term excellence of our calling in the future. By investing in leadership development throughout health provider professions and health service organisations, that challenge can be met and our patients' lives improved.

References

Introduction

1 Dickens C. *A Tale of Two Cities*. Project Gutenberg Literary Archive Foundation; posted 28 November 2009 (last updated 23 January 2011). Available at: www.gutenberg.org/ebooks/98 (accessed 28 August 2011).

2 Bootle R. Why most things keep getting better – and a few get worse. *Daily Telegraph*. 28 August 2011; B2.

3 Morris I. *Why the West Rules – For Now: the patterns of history, and what they reveal about the future*. Nuneaton, UK: Profile; 2010.

4 Greenfield S. *Tomorrow's People: how 21st century technology is changing the way we think and feel*. 2nd ed. London: Penguin Books; 2004.

5 Henry CM. Beyond 2000: the next pharmaceutical century. Available at: www2.uah.es/farmamol/The%20Pharmaceutical%20Century/Ch10.html (accessed 20 April 2008).

6 United Nations. *United Nations Millennium Declaration*. New York, NY: United Nations; September 2000. Available at: www.un.org/millennium/declaration/ares552e.htm (accessed 20 April 2001).

7 UN Millennium Project, Task Force on Child Health and Maternal Health. *Who's Got the Power? Transforming health systems for women and children*. London: Earthscan; 2005.

8 Joy B. Why the future doesn't need us. *Wired*. April 2000; (8.04).

Chapter 1: Key drivers of change

9 Kurowska K with Whaley P. Demographic change and an ageing population: the policy context. Available at: www.ncl.ac.uk/iah/research/programmes/documents/DEMOGRAPHICCHANGEANDANAGEINGPOPULATION.pdf (accessed 20 June 2011).

10 Lueddeke GR. *History of Medicine and Medical Education in Britain: from bad to good medicine?* [interactive lecture series]: Southampton: School of Medicine, University of Southampton; 2005.

11 World Health Organization. *The World Health Report 2006: working together for health*. Geneva: WHO: 2006. Available at: www.who.int/whr/2006/en/ (accessed 15 June 2011).

12 United Nations. Millennium development goals reports. Available at: www.un.org/millenniumgoals/reports.shtml (accessed 20 June 2011).

13 World Health Organization. *Closing the Gap in a Generation: health equity through action on the social determinants of health*. Geneva: WHO; 2008.

14 Martin D. The children eating their way to cancer: expert warns of obesity timebomb. *Mail Online*. 4 February 2009. Available at: www.dailymail.co.uk/health/article-1135427/The-children-eating-way-cancer-Expert-warns-obesity-timebomb.html (accessed 15 September 2010).

15 National Heart, Lung, and Blood Institute. Calculate your body mass index [calculation tool]. Available at: www.nhlbisupport.com/bmi/ (accessed 28 July 2011).

References

16 Hive Health Media. *World Obesity Stats: 2010 and beyond*. Hive Health Media; September 2010. Available at: www.hivehealthmedia.com/world-obesity-stats-2010/ (accessed 27 February 2011).

17 Organisation for Economic Co-operation and Development (OECD). *Obesity and the Economics of Prevention: fit not fat*. Paris: OECD; 2010. Available at: www.oecd.org/document/31/0,3746,en_2649_33929_45999775_1_1_1_1,00.html (accessed 20 August 2011).

18 Trust for America's Health (TFAH). *F as in Fat: how obesity threatens America's future 2011*. Washington, DC: TFAH; July 2011. Available at: http://healthyamericans.org/report/88/ (accessed 24 August 2011).

19 Public Health Agency of Canada (PHAC) and Canadian Institute for Health Information. *Obesity in Canada*. Ontario: PHAC; June 2011. Available at: www.phac-aspc.gc.ca/hp-ps/hl-mvs/oic-oac/index-eng.php (accessed 28 August 2011).

20 Mara D. *New Obesity Report Says World is Fatter, Rounder, Less Productive*. Bonn: Deutsche Welle; February 2011. Available at: www.dw-world.de/dw/article/0,,14818710,00.html (accessed 24 August 2011).

21 Bates C. Fat Britain: tackling the obesity epidemic. *Mail Online*. Available at: www.dailymail.co.uk/health/article-301419/Fat-Britain-Tackling-obesity-epidemic.html (accessed 26 October 2011).

22 Monash Obesity and Diabetes Institute, Monash University. *Facts and Figures: obesity in Australia*. Available at: www.modi.monash.edu.au/obesity-facts-figures/obesity-in-australia/ (accessed 26 September 2011).

23 China on msnbc.com. *Richer but Fatter? China weight loss camps battle bulge*. msnbc.com; [updated 26 August 2011]. Available at: www.msnbc.msn.com/id/44283668/ns/world_news-asia_pacific/t/richer-fatter-china-weight-loss-camps-battle-bulge/ (accessed 24 October 2011).

24 National Obesity Observatory. *International Comparisons of Obesity Prevalence*. Available at: www.noo.org.uk/NOO_about_obesity/international/ (accessed 20 October 2011).

25 Macera CA; Division of Nutrition and Physical Activity National Center for Chronic Disease Prevention and Health Promotion, Centers for Disease Control and Prevention. *Promoting Healthy Eating and Physical Activity for a Healthier Nation*. Centers for Disease Control and Prevention. Available at: www.cdc.gov/healthyyouth/publications/pdf/PP-Ch7.pdf (accessed 25 July 2011).

26 European Association for the Study of Obesity (EASO). *EASO Strategic Plan 2010–2012*. Middlesex: EASO; 2010. Available at: www.easo.org/documents/EASOStrategicPlan-WebsiteVersion.pdf (accessed 29 August 2011).

27 Frenk J. *Editorial Reviews of Obesity and the Economics of Prevention: fit not fat (2010)*. Paris: OECD. Available at: www.oecd.org/document/34/0,3746,en_2649_33929_46047202_1_1_1_1,00.html (accessed 25 August 2011).

28 McKee M. *Editorial Reviews of Obesity and the Economics of Prevention: fit not fat (2010)*. Paris: OECD. Available at: www.oecd.org/document/11/0,3746,en_2649_33929_46047243_1_1_1_1,00.html (accessed 25 February 2011).

29 Tobin D. Cars adapt to fit our bulging bodywork. *Sunday Star Times*. 23 October 2011. Available at: www.timesplus.co.uk/sto/?login=false&url=http%3A%2F%2Fwww.thesundaytimes.co.uk%2Fsto%2Fnews%2Fuk_news%2FSociety%2Farticle804787.ece (accessed 24 October 2011).

30 Cordain L. Cereal grains: humanity's double-edged sword. *World Rev Nutr Diet*. 1999; **84**: 19–73.

31 Ferriss T. How to keep feces out of your bloodstream (or lose 10 pounds in 14 days). *The Blog of Tim Ferriss*. Available at: www.fourhourworkweek.com/blog/2010/09/19/paleo-diet-solution/ (accessed 20 June 2011).

32 Crayon R. The Paleolithic diet and its modern implications [interview with Dr Loren Cordain]. Available at: www.becomehealthynow.com/article/carbs/11 (accessed 20 March 2007).

33 Food and Agriculture Organization (FAO). *Staple Foods: what do people eat?* Available at: www. fao.org/docrep/u8480e/u8480e07.htm (accessed 10 July 2011).

34 Lindeberg S, Jönsson T, Granfeldt Y, *et al*. A Palaeolithic diet improves glucose tolerance more than a Mediterranean-like diet in individuals with ischaemic heart disease. *Diabetologia*. 2007; **50**(9): 1795–807.

35 *Paleolithic Diet in the Treatment of Diabetes Type 2 in Primary Health Care*. ClinicalTrials. gov; 13 February 2007 [updated 13 May 2008]. Available at: http://clinicaltrials.gov/ct2/show/ NCT00435240 (accessed 20 September 2009).

36 World Hunger Education Service. *2011 World Hunger and Poverty Facts and Statistics (2011)*. Washington, DC: World Hunger Education Service. Available at: www.worldhunger.org/ articles/Learn/world%20hunger%20facts%202002.htm (accessed 20 June 2011).

37 International Food Policy Research Institute, Concern Worldwide, Welthungerhilfe. *Global Hunger Index 2010: malnutrition amongst young children is the face of worldwide hunger*. Deutsche Welthungerhilfe eV; October 2010. Available at: www.welthungerhilfe.de/ghi2010. html (accessed 20 October 2011).

38 Global Sherpa. World food prices hit record high. *Global Sherpa*. 4 February 2011. Available at: www.globalsherpa.org/food-prices-crisis (accessed 14 March 2011).

39 Sisson M. The definitive guide to grains. *Mark's Daily Apple*. Available at: www.marksdaily apple.com/definitive-guide-grains/ (accessed 25 August 2011).

40 ACS Publications. *The Pharmaceutical Century: 10 decades of drug discovery 1990s*. Available at: www2.uah.es/farmamol/The%20Pharmaceutical%20Century/index.html (accessed 18 October 2010).

41 Diabetes UK. *Diabetes Rates in the UK Soar to Nearly 3m*. London: Diabetes UK; October 2011. Available at: www.diabetes.org.uk/About_us/News_Landing_Page/Diabetes-rates-in-the-UK-soar-to-nearly-3m/ (accessed 28 October 2011).

42 Borland S. Diabetes rises by 50% in five years. *Daily Mail*. 27 October 2011: 13.

43 Society of Actuaries. The economic cost of obesity. *Insurance Journal*. 11 January 2011. Available at: www.insurancejournal.com/news/national/2011/01/11/180022.htm (accessed 20 April 2011).

44 Finkelstein EA, DiBonaventura MD, Burgess SM, *et al*. The costs of obesity in the workplace. *J Occup Environ Med*. 2010; **52**(10): 971–6.

45 Reinberg S. Almost 10 percent of U.S. medical costs tied to obesity. *ABC News*. July 2009. Available at: http://abcnews.go.com/Health/Healthday/story?id=8184975&page=1 (accessed 27 August 2011).

46 HM Treasury. NHS – UK public spending. Available at: www.ukpublicspending.co.uk/ uk_year2010_0.html%3C/uk_health_care_budget_2010_1.html (accessed 3 June 2011).

47 Royal College of Nursing. *UK2 2011 Budget Impacts Health Research*. Available at: www.rcn. org.uk/development/researchanddevelopment/newsevents/research_policy_and_practice/ uk_2011_budget_impacts_health_research (accessed 20 October 2011).

48 Ozuah PO. Undergraduate medical education: thoughts on future challenges. *BMC Med Educ*. 2002; **2**: 8.

49 Charles J. *Key Influences on Future Trends in Healthcare*. Cardiff: National Public Health Service for Wales; 2008.

50 Centre for Global Health Policy and Innovation Blog. Health care spending: large differences, unequal results. WordPress.com. Available at: http://increasingaccesstomedicines.wordpress. com/ (accessed 20 June 2011).

51 Hand R. NatGeo shows healthcare spending vs. life expectancy. Available at: www.vizworld.com/ 2010/01/natgeo-shows-health-care-spending-life-expectancy/ (accessed 20 August 2011).

52 Buttonwood. Buttonwood's notebook: healthcare spending and life expectancy; sick note. *The Economist*. 18 March 2011. Available at: www.economist.com/blogs/buttonwood/2011/03/ healthcare_spending_and_life_expectancy (accessed 26 May 2011).

References

53 Leon DA. Trends in European life expectancy: a salutary view. *Int J Epidemiol*. 2011; **40**(2): 271–7.

54 Davis K, Schoen C, Stremikis K. *Mirror, Mirror On The Wall: how the performance of the U.S. healthcare system compares internationally: 2010 update*. New York, NY: The Commonwealth Fund; June 2010. Available at: www.commonwealthfund.org/~/media/Files/Publications/Fund%20Report/2010/Jun/1400_Davis_Mirror_Mirror_on_the_wall_2010.pdf (accessed 20 February 2011).

55 Flier JS. Health 'reform' gets a failing grade. *Wall Street Journal*. 17 November 2009. Available at: http://online.wsj.com/article/SB10001424052748704431804574539581994054014.html (accessed 20 December 2009).

56 Frenk J, Chen L, Bhutta ZA, *et al*. Health professionals for a new century: transforming education to strengthen health systems in an interdependent world. *Lancet*. 2010; **376**(9756): 1923–58.

57 Smyth C. Patients face longer wait as NHS 'slips backwards' under coalition. *The Times*. 19 August 2011: 11.

58 Country. Long emergency room wait time in Canada provokes man to take drastic measures. *Why My Country Sucks: real stories from around the globe*; 5 March 2011. Available at: http://whymycountrysucks.com/north-america/canada/long-emergency-room-wait-time-in-canada-provokes-man-to-take-drastic-measures/#ixzz1aMve6xT0 (accessed 10 June 2011).

59 Arnst C. The doctor will see you – in three months. *Business Week*. 9 July 2007. Available at: www.businessweek.com/magazine/content/07_28/b4042072.htm (accessed 10 June 2010).

60 Kerin L. No substantial change in hospital waiting times. *ABC News*. 30 November 2010. Available at: www.abc.net.au/news/2010-11-30/no-substantial-change-in-hospital-waiting-times/2357096 (accessed 25 January 2011).

61 World Health Organization. *The World Health Report 2008: primary health care (now more than ever)*. Geneva: WHO; 2008. Available at: www.who.int/whr/2008/en/index.html (accessed 12 May 2009).

62 Thomas DJ. A caring state of mind and the time to look after patients. Letters to the Editor. *The Times*. 23 September 2011: 35.

63 Cavendish C. Nurse training has eroded the caring ethos. *The Times*. 22 September 2011: 27.

64 Borland S. Wait 3 weeks to see GP. *Daily Mail*. 21 September 2011: 13.

65 Smyth C. Trust trains its own nurses to nurture better 'attitudes'. *The Times*. 4 October 2011: 11.

66 Health News. Low health literacy linked to higher risk of death and more emergency room visits and hospitalisations. *Health Blogs*. 30 May 2011. Available at: http://healthblogs.org/2011/05/30/low-health-literacy-linked-to-higher-risk-of-death-and-more-emergency-room-visits-and-hospitalizations/ (accessed 10 June 2011).

67 Molina HealthCare, California Academy of Family Physicians. *'I Hear You Talking, But I Don't Understand You!' Medical jargon and clear communication*. San Francisco, CA: CAFP; April 2004. Available at: www.familydocs.org/assets/Multicultural_Health/MedicalJargon.pdf (accessed 15 June 2011).

68 US Department of Health and Human Services, Office of Disease Prevention and Health Promotion. *National Action Plan to Improve Health Literacy*. Washington, DC: US Department of Health and Human Services; 2010.

69 Rossiter A. *The Future of Healthcare*. London: Social Market Foundation; 2007. Available at: http://smf.co.uk/assets/filrs/publications?Thr%20Future20of%20Healthcare.pdf (accessed 20 February 2009).

70 Department of Health. *Future Health Care Trends: an overview*. Available at: www.national leadershipnetwork.otg/public/NLN+future trends (accessed 20 June 2009).

71 Department of Health; David Colin-Thomé, National Director for Primary Care. *Keeping It Personal: clinical case for change*. London: Department of Health; 2007. Available at: www.dh.gov.uk/en/Publicationsandstatistics/Publications/PublicationsPolicyAndGuidance/DH_065094 (accessed 19 July 2009).

72 Smith R. *Globalisation of the Empowered Health Care Consumer* [PowerPoint]. Available at: www.resources.bmj.com/files/talks/global.ppt 9 (accessed 2 May 2007).

73 Greenhalgh T, Hinder S, Stramer K, *et al*. Adoption, non-adoption, and abandonment of a personal electronic health record: case study of HealthSpace. *BMJ*. 2010; **341**: c5814.

74 Lloyd-Williams D. *Looking to the Future: the added value of ehealth*. Available at: www.silicon bridge.co.uk/art_future_ehealth.html (accessed 25 June 2011).

75 European Parkinson's Disease Association. *OECD Publishes Report on Providing and Paying for Long-Term Care*. London: EPDA: May 2011. Available at: www.epda.eu.com/news/2011-05-18-oecd/ (accessed 15 June 2011).

76 Lueddeke GR. The changing landscape of UK medical education: trends and future possibilities. Presented at Wessex Deanery Faculty Conference, 2010 April 9; Hampshire, UK.

77 Jacobs F. *The Patients Per Doctor Map of the World*. Big Think; October 2007. Available at: http://bigthink.com/ideas/21237 (accessed 8 May 2011).

78 Dayrit MM, Dolea C, Dreesch N. *Adressing the HRH crisis in countries: how far have we gone? What can we expect to achieve by 2015?* Available at: www.scielo.org.pe/pdf/rins/v28n2/a27v28n2.pdf (accessed 29 November 2011).

79 Family Care Foundation. *If the World Were a Village of 100 People*. Available at: www.family care.org/special-interest/if-the-world-were-a-village-of-100-people/ (accessed 15 July 2010).

80 Chan M. Margaret Chan puts primary health care centre stage at WHO. *The Lancet*. 2008; **37**(9627): 1811.

81 Schimpff S. *The Future of Medicine: megatrends in healthcare that will improve your quality of life*. Nashville, TN: Thomas Nelson; 2007.

82 Bostridge M. *Florence Nightingale: the making of an icon*. New York, NY: Farrar, Straus & Giroux; 2008.

83 Yanchick VA. Multidisciplinary education: a challenge for pharmacy education. *Am J Pharm Educ*. 2004; **68**(3): 1–2.

84 House of Commons Health Committee. *The Victoria Climbié Inquiry Report*. London: The Stationery Office; June 2003. Available at: www.publications.parliament.uk/pa/cm200203/cmselect/cmhealth/570/570.pdf (accessed 20 January 2004).

85 Centre for the Advancement of Interprofessional Education (CAIPE). *Interprofessional Education: a definition*. Available at: www.caipe.org.uk/about-us/defining-ipe/ (accessed 20 May 2011).

86 Thistlethwaite J, Barr H, Gilbert J. Transforming health professionals' education. *The Lancet*. 2011; **377**(9773): 1236.

87 O'Halloran C, Humphris D. *Common Learning in Health and Socialcare: the new generation curriculum model* [PowerPoint]. Available at: www.commonlearning.net/docs/news/COHalloran%20presentation%20UBC%20May%202004.ppt (accessed 10 June 2004).

88 Jackson P. *Developing and Delivering Undergraduate Interprofessional Learning: a collaboration*. Available at: www.uhmlg.ac.uk/documents/jackson-summer2011.ppt (accessed 20 November 2011).

89 Naylor, D, Serwadda D, Meleis A, *et al*. Launch panels. Panel 1: transforming the learning process [Harvard launch of health commission report]. Available at: www.healthprofessionals 21.org/index.php/the-report/launch-event (accessed 25 January 2011).

90 Taskforce on Multidisciplinary Learning and Team Teaching. *Final Report*. Available at: www. umich.edu/pres/init/init3.php (accessed 29 December 2005).

91 Davidson C. So last century. *The Times Higher Education*. 28 April 2011.

92 Bainbridge L. Interprofessional education for interprofessional practice: will future health care providers embrace collaboration as one answer to improved quality of care? *UBCMJ*. 2010; **2**(1): 9–10.

93 Daly G. Understanding the barriers to multiprofessional collaboration. *Nurs Times*. 2004; **100**(9): 78–9.

94 Leathard A. *Interprofessional Collaboration: from policy to practice in health and social care.* Sussex, UK: Psychology Press; 2003.

95 Association of Faculties of Medicine of Canada. *Accreditation of Interprofessional Health Education (AIPHE): principles and practices for integrating interprofessional education into the accreditation standards for six health professions in Canada.* Available at: www.afmc.ca/projects-aiphe-e.php (accessed 15 July 2011).

96 Canadian Interprofessional Health Collaborative. *A National Competency Framework for Interprofessional Collaboration.* Vancouver, BC: CIHC; February 2010. Available at: www.cihc.ca/files/CIHC_IPCompetencies_Feb1210.pdf (accessed 19 August 2011).

97 NHS Institute for Innovation and Improvement. *Medical Leadership Competency Framework.* Available at: www.institute.nhs.uk/assessment_tool/general/medical_leadership_competency_framework_-_homepage.html (accessed 19 September 2007).

98 World Health Organization. *Framework for Action on Interprofessional Education and Collaborative Practice.* Geneva: WHO; 2010.

99 Irvine D. Medicine beyond 2000: trust me I am (still) a doctor. *Ulster Med J.* 1998; **67**(Suppl 1): 103–6.

Chapter 2: National reviews of medical education

100 Australian Government Department of Education, Employment and Workplace Relations. *What Makes for Success in Medical Education? Synthesis report.* Commonwealth of Australia; 2008. Available at: www.deewr.gov.au/HigherEducation/Publications/HEReports/Documents/SynthesisReport.pdf (accessed 15 June 2011).

101 Association of Faculties of Medicine of Canada (AFMC). *The Future of Medical Education in Canada (FMEC): a collective vision for MD education (2010).* Available at: www.afmc.ca/fmec/pdf/collective_vision.pdf (accessed 15 August 2011).

102 Cooke M, Irby D, O'Brien B. *Educating Physicians: a call for reform of medical school and residency.* San Francisco, CA: Jossey-Bass; 2010.

103 Josiah Macy Jr Foundation. *Ensuring an Effective Physician Workforce for America: recommendations for an accountable graduate medical education system.* New York, NY: Josiah Macy Jr Foundation; February 2011. Available at: www.josiahmacyfoundation.org/news/entry/health-care-leaders-gme-system-needs-to-better-align-with-patient-needs (accessed 29 August 2011).

104 Josiah Macy Jr Foundation. *Ensuring an Effective Physician Workforce for the United States: recommendations for reforming graduate medical education to meet the needs of the public.* New York, NY: Josiah Macy Jr Foundation; 2011. Available at: www.aocoohns.org/wp-content/uploads/2011/11/GME-MACY-Article-September-2011.pdf (accessed 15 November 2011).

105 American College of Physicians (ACP). *'Aligning GME Policy with the Nation's Health Care Workforce Needs' Policy Paper Released by Physicians.* Philadelphia, PA: ACP; 7 September 2011. Available at: www.acponline.org/pressroom/gme_policy.htm (accessed 16 October 2011).

106 Kanter SL. Proposals to strengthen the link between medical education and better health for individuals and populations. *Acad Med.* 2011; **86**(11): 1329.

107 General Medical Council. *GMC Education Strategy 2011–2013.* London: GMC; 2010.

108 General Medical Council. *The State of Medical Education and Practice 2011.* Available at: www.gmc-uk.org/State_of_medicine_Final_web.pdf_44213427.pdf (accessed 20 September 2011).

109 Corrigan P. Why the Tories will have to close hospitals (and so would Labour if they were still in power) from Blair's health guru. *Mail Online.* 18 September 2011. Available at: www.dailymail.co.uk/debate/article-2038505/Why-Tories-close-hospitals-Labour-power.html (accessed 20 September 2011).

110 Keogh B. NHS has no future if we perpetuate mediocrity. *The Times.* 23 June 2011: 24.

111 Burness Communications. *Macy Foundation Report Calls for Sweeping Graduate Medical Education Reforms.* Press Release. New York, NY: Macy Foundation; Thursday 8 September

2011. Available at: www.eurekalert.org/pub_releases/2011-09/bc-mfr090811.php (accessed 15 October 2011).

112 Cavendish C. NHS: the Cavendish report. Part 1. *The Times*. 25 May 2011: 11.

113 Hamberger B. Surgery in Sweden. *Arch Surg*. 1998; **133**(3): 323–6. Available at: http://archsurg.ama-assn.org/cgi/reprint/133/3/323.pdf (accessed 18 July 2011).

114 American Academy of Family Physicians (AAFP). *Family Physician Workforce Reform: recommendations of the American Academy of Family Physicians*. Available at: www.aafp.org/online/en/home/policy/policies/w/workforce.html (accessed 10 August 2011).

115 Lee PT, Kerry VB, Stone VE, *et al*. Transforming health professionals' education. *The Lancet*. 2011; **377**(9773): 1235.

116 Zurayk H, Cohen J, Henney J, *et al*. Launch panels. Panel 2: reforming educational institutions [Harvard launch of health commission report]. Available at: http://healthprofessionals21.org/index.php/the-report/launch-event/launch-panels (accessed 15 July 2011).

Chapter 3: Educational priorities in medical education

117 Lueddeke GR. Curriculum matters: building capacity for strategic change in UK higher education. *IJSCM*. 2010; **2**(1): 18–31.

118 Kuiper RA, Pesut DJ. Promoting cognitive and metacognitive reflective reasoning skills in nursing practice: self-regulated learning theory. *J Adv Nurs*. 2004; **45**(4): 381–91.

119 Johnson M. 20th century medical education won't be enough, experts say. *Journal Sentinel*. 30 November 2010. Available at: www.jsonline.com/blogs/news/111042774.html (accessed 17 May 2011).

120 The Johns Hopkins Health System. *Celebrating the Contributions of William Osler*. Available at: www.medicalarchives.jhmi.edu/osler/biography.htm (accessed 20 May 2011).

121 Bonner TN. *Iconoclast: Abraham Flexner and a life in learning*. Baltimore, MD: The Johns Hopkins University Press; 2002.

122 Duclaux E. *Pasteur: the history of a mind*. Palo Alto, CA: Stanford University; 1920.

123 Brock TD. *Robert Koch: a life in medicine and bacteriology*. Washington, DC: American Society for Microbiology; 1999.

124 Osler W. *The Principles and Practice of Medicine: designed for the use of practitioners and students of medicine*. 1st ed. New York, NY: D Appleton; 1901.

125 Flexner A. *Medical education in the United States and Canada: a report to the Carnegie Foundation for the Advancement of Teaching* [Carnegie Foundation Bulletin No. 4]. New York, NY: Carnegie Foundation for the Advancement of Teaching; 1910.

126 Chambers DA. Flexner at 100: a perspective. *Perspect Biol Med*. 2011; **54**(1): 3–7.

127 Crisp N, Evans T, Garcia P, *et al*. Launch panels. Panel 3: Local adaptability in a global world. [Harvard launch of health commission report]. Available at: http://healthprofessionals21.org/index.php/the-report/launch-event/launch-panels (accessed 15 July 2011).

128 Holmboe E, Ginsburg S, Bernabeo E. The rotational approach to medical education: time to confront our assumptions? *Med Educ*. 2011; **45**(1): 69–80.

129 Smith R. *The Future of Health Care* [PowerPoint]. Available at: resources.bmj.com/files/talks/futurepoints.ppt (accessed 2 May 2007).

130 Hammond P. The NHS can learn a lot from India … and Scotland. *The Times*. 5 September 2011: 26.

131 Bennet D. *Expanding the Knowledge Paradigm*. Available at: http://mountainquestinstitute.com/Expand%20the%20Kn%20Paradigm%202006.pdf (accessed 16 May 2007).

132 Inglis A. Theories of learning in educational development: relocating the paradigm divide. *Open Learning*. 1996; **11**(2): 28–37.

133 Lueddeke GR. Toward a constructivist framework for guiding change and innovation in higher education. *J High Educ*. 1999; **70**(3): 235–60.

134 Tweed R, Lehman D. Learning considered within a cultural context: Confucian and Socratic approaches. *Am Psychol*. 2002; **57**(2): 89–99.

References

135 Ozmon H, Craver S. *Philosophical Foundations of Education*. 8th ed. New Jersey: Prentice Hall; 2007.

136 Schön DA. *The Reflective Practitioner: how professionals think in action*. San Francisco, CA: Jossey-Bass; 1987.

137 Senge P. The academy as a learning community. In: Lucas AF, editor. *Leading Academic Change: essential roles for department chairs*. San Francisco, CA: Jossey-Bass; 2000. pp. 275–300.

138 Kuhn T. *The Structure of Scientific Revolution*. Chicago: University of Chicago Press; 1962.

139 Bennett M. *The Myers-Briggs Personality Indicator*. Ventana Center for Psychotherapy. Available at: www.ventanacenter.com/articlesbackground_003.htm (accessed 27 August 2006).

140 Lievens F, Coetsier P, De Fruyt F, *et al*. Medical students' personality characteristics and academic performance: a five-factor model perspective. *Med Educ*. 2002: **36**(11): 1050–6.

141 Stilwell NA, Wallick MM, Thal SE, *et al*. Myers-Briggs type and medical specialty choice: a new look at an old question. *Teach Learn Med*. 2000; **12**(1): 14–20.

142 Katz J. Myers-Briggs personality type of medical students (2010). Available at: www.personalitydesk.com/blog/myers-briggs-personality-type-medical-students#axzz1ke H1qaLH (accessed 28 August 2011).

143 Dall'Alba G, Sandberg J. Unveiling professional development: a critical review of stage models. *Rev Educ Res*. 2006; **76**(3): 383–412. Available at: http://rer.sagepub.com/content/76/3/383 (accessed 21 May 2011).

Chapter 4: Medical education: learning systems review and development

144 Stanford Centre for Opportunity Policy in Education. *Reframing student outcomes to develop 21st century skills: knowledge brief*. Stanford, CA: SCOPE.

145 Gruppen LD, Mangrulkar RS, Kaolars JC. *Competency-Based Education in the Health Professions: implications for improving global health*. 2010. Available at: http://healthprofes sionals21.org/docs/CompBasedEd.pdf (accessed 18 February 2010).

146 Albanese MA, Mejicano G, Mullan P, *et al*. Defining characteristics of educational competencies. *Med Educ*. 2008; **42**(3): 248–55.

147 Thier SO. *Talk at the Launch of the Commission Report* [Harvard launch of health commission report]. 30 November 2010. Available at: www.healthprofessionals21.org/index.php/the-report/comments/27-talk-at-the-launch-of-the-commission-report-november-30-2010 (accessed 25 January 2011).

148 Rubin P. Junior doctors need supervised experience of many patients. Letters to the Editor. *The Times*. 13 September 2010.

149 World Health Organization. *Increasing Access to Health Workers in Remote and Rural Areas through Improved Retention: global policy recommendations*. Geneva: WHO; 2010.

150 Lueddeke GR. *Meeting Employer Needs: applying the DACUM approach to undergraduate and postgraduate curriculum design*. Seminar for School of Education; 17 September 2010; Southampton, UK: University of Southampton.

151 UNESCO-UNEVOC. *Dacum*. Available at: www.unevoc.unesco.org/tvetipedia.0.html?&tx_ drwiki_pi1[keyword]=DACUM (accessed 20 April 2011).

152 CareerOneStop. *Competency Model Clearinghouse* [online tutorial]. Available at: www. careeronestop.org/competencymodel/Tutorials/SiteTutorial.htm (accessed 20 May 2011).

Chapter 5: Case examples: learning systems implementation

153 Siega-Sur JLJ. *The UPM-SHS: where health workers are trained to stay and serve*. Available at: www.up.edu.ph/oldforum/2005/Jul-Aug05/UPM-SHS.html (accessed 7 December 2011).

154 Training for Health Equity Network: THEnet. *UPS SHS Leyte* (University of the Philippines School of Health Sciences, Leyte). Available at: www.thenetcommunity.org/our-members-a-partners/joomla-license/university-of-the-phillipines-shs.html (accessed 7 December 2011).

155 Lueddeke GR. *Working with Learning Outcomes that 'Motivate and Matter'*. Workshop, University of Southampton, UK; 5 September 2011.

156 Beaumont R, Spencer J. *Learning Outcomes: a practical guide*. 28 November 2005. Available at: www.fhi.rcsed.ac.uk/rbeaumont/virtualclassroom/chap21/s1/outc6.pdf (accessed 29 October 2008).

157 Federation of the Royal Colleges of Physicians (FRCP). *Generic Curriculum for the Medical Specialties*. 4th ed. London: FRCP; 2010. Available at: www.gmc-uk.org/generic_curriculum ___may_07.pdf_30291352.pdf (accessed 19 February 2011).

158 Joint Royal Colleges of Physicians Training Board (JRCPTB). *Specialty Training Framework for Core Medical Training*. London: JRCPTB; August 2009. Available at: www.gmc-uk. org/2009_CMT_FINAL.pdf_36112862.pdf (accessed 19 February 2011).

159 Fish D, Coles C. *Medical Education: developing a curriculum for practice*. Berkshire, UK: Open University Press; 2005.

160 Thompson R. Patients at risk in our hospitals. *Independent*. 9 September 2011. Available at: www.independent.co.uk/opinion/letters/letters-patients-at-risk-in-our-hospitals-2351549. html (accessed 23 September 2011).

161 Battles JB. Quality and safety by design. *Qual Saf Health Care*. 2006: **15**(Suppl 1); i1–13.

162 Nutton V, Porter R. *The History of Medical Education in Britain*. Amsterdam: Rodopi; 1995.

163 Shorter E. *Doctors and Their Patients: a social history*. London: Transaction Publishers; 2007.

164 Brimelow A. GMC says more support needed for overseas doctors in UK. *BBC News*. 16 September 2011. Available at: www.bbc.co.uk/news/health-14921313 (accessed 19 September 2011).

165 Boyer Commission on Educating Undergraduates in the Research University. *Reinventing Undergraduate Education: a blueprint for America's research universities (1998)*. Available at: http://naples.cc.sunysb.edu/Pres/boyer.nsf/ (accessed 12 February 2001).

166 Lueddeke GR. Applying a constructivist framework to strategic change and innovation in research-intensive universities. *International Journal of Knowledge, Culture & Change Management*. 2007; **6**(7): 198–213.

167 Diaz C. Australian Awards for University Teaching – 2011: citation for outstanding contributions to student learning. Available at: www.altc.edu.au/award-outstanding-contributions-recipient-2011-associate-professor-diaz (accessed 15 August 2011).

168 Biggs J. *Aligning Teaching for Constructive Learning*. Available at: www.heacademy.ac.uk/ assets/documents/resources/resourcedatabase/id477_aligning_teaching_for_constructing_ learning.pdf (accessed 23 May 2003).

169 Shellard D. Abandon comfort all ye who enter this arena of challenge and renewal. *The Times Higher Education*. 17 June 2010. Available at: www.timeshighereducation.co.uk/story. asp?storycode=412073 (accessed 30 June 2010).

Chapter 6: Medical education and the management of change

170 Mortensen L, Malling B, Ringsted C, *et al*. What is the impact of a national postgraduate medical specialist education reform on the daily clinical training 3.5 years after implementation? A questionnaire survey. *BMC Med Educ*. 2010; **10**: 46.

171 Wooton D. *Bad Medicine: doctors doing harm since Hippocrates*. Oxford: Oxford University Press; 2007.

172 Bolman L, Deal T. *Reframing Organizations: artistry, choice, and leadership*. San Francisco, CA: Jossey-Bass; 2003.

173 Schein E. *Organizational Culture and Leadership: a dynamic view*. 2nd ed. San Francisco, CA: Jossey-Bass; 1992.

174 Mannion R, McDonald R, Fulup N, *et al*. *Changing Management Cultures and Organisational Performance in the NHS (OC2)*. Research report produced for the National Institute for Health Research Service Delivery and Organisation programme. London: Queen's Printer and Controller of HMSO; 2010.

References

175 Bergquist W. *The Four Cultures of the Academy*. San Francisco, CA: Jossey-Bass; 1992.

176 Lester S. *Learning for the 21st Century*. Available at: www.sld.demon.co.uk/lrg21st.pdf (accessed 21 June 2000).

177 Birnbaum R. *How Colleges Work: the cybernetics of academic organization and leadership*. San Francisco, CA: Jossey-Bass; 1988.

178 Olssen M. Radical constructivism and its failings: anti-realism and individualism. *Brit J Educ Stud*. 1996; **44**(3): 275–95.

179 Jonassen D, Davidson M, Collins M, *et al*. Constructivism and computer-mediated communication in distance education. *AJDE*. 1995; **9**(2): 7–26.

180 Savery J, Duffy T. Problem-based learning: an instructional model and its constructivist framework. *Educ Technol*. 1995; **35**(5): 31–8.

181 Bensimon E, Neumann A. *Redesigning Collegiate Leadership: teams and teamwork in higher education*. Baltimore, MD: The Johns Hopkins University Press; 1994.

182 Davies J. The evolution of university responses to financial reduction. *Higher Educ Manage*. 1997; **9**(1): 127–40.

183 Hargreaves A, Lieberman A, Fullan M, *et al*., editors. *Second International Handbook of Educational Change*. New York, NY: Springer Publishing; 2010.

184 Hargreaves A. Renewal in the age of paradox. *Educ Leadership*. 1995; **52**(7): 14–19.

185 Willis J. A recursive, reflective instructional design model based on constructivist interpretive theory. *Educ Technol*. 1995; **35**(6): 5–23.

186 Fullan M, Miles M. Getting reform right: what works and what doesn't. *Phi Delta Kappan*. 1992; **73**(1): 744–52.

187 Davies HTO. Understanding organisational culture in reforming the National Health Service. *J R Soc Med*. 2002; **95**(3): 140–2.

188 Duderstadt J. *A University for the 21st Century*. Ann Arbor: University of Michigan; 2000.

189 Lindquist J. *Strategies for Change*. Berkeley, CA: Pacific Sounding Press; 1978.

190 Gaff J. *Toward Faculty Renewal: advances in faculty, institutional and organisational development*. San Francisco, CA: Jossey-Bass; 1975.

191 Smollan RK, Sayers JG. Organizational culture, organizational change and emotions: a qualitative study. *J Change Management*. 2009; **9**(4): 435–57.

192 Knight P, Trowler P. Departmental-level cultures and the improvement of learning and teaching. *Stud High Educ*. 2000; **25**(1): 69–83.

193 Massy W, Wilger A, Colbeck C. Overcoming 'hollowed' collegiality. *Change*. 1994: **26**(4): 10–20.

194 Stok-Koch L, Bolhuis S, Koopmans R. Identifying factors that influence workplace learning in postgraduate medical education. *Educ Health (Abingdon)*. 2007: **20**(1): 8.

195 Academy of Medical Educators. *Professional Standards*. Available at: http://medicaleducators.org/index.cfm/profession/profstandards/ (accessed 10 October 2010).

196 Bligh J, Brice J. Leadership in medical education. *BMJ*. 2010; **340**: c2351. Available at: www.bmj.com/content/340/bmj.c2351.full (accessed 30 May 2011).

197 Collins-Nakai R. Leadership in medicine. *Mcgill J Med*. 2006; **9**(1): 68–73.

198 Souba WW. Building our future: a plea for leadership. *World J Surg*. 2004; **28**(5): 445–50.

199 Lao Tzu. Available at: www.goodreads.com/author/quotes/2622245.Lao_Tzu (accessed 15 July 2011).

Chapter 7: The physician–patient contract

200 Duffin J. *History of Medicine: a scandalously short introduction*. 3rd ed. Toronto: University of Toronto Press; 2004.

201 Smith R. *Where Are the Limits of Medicine: are we turning the whole world into patients?* [PowerPoint]. Available at: resources.bmj.com/files/talks/santiago.ppt (accessed 2 May 2007).

202 Maeshiro R, Koo D, Keck CW. Integration of public health into medical education: an introduction to the supplement. *Am J Prev Med*. 2011; **41**(4 Suppl 3): S145–8.

203 Prescott JE. Exploring the context: contemporary medical education. *Am J Prev Med*. 2011; **41**(4): S160–3.

204 Dahlstrom J, Dorai-Raj A, McGill D, *et al*. What motivates senior clinicians to teach medical students? *BMC Med Educ*. 2005; **5**: 27. Available at: www.biomedcentral.com/1472-6920/5/27 (accessed 20 September 2007).

205 Kolata G. When the doctor is in, but you wish he weren't. *NY Times*. 30 November 2005. Available at: www.anapsid.org/cnd/support/rushdocs.html (accessed 20 April 2010).

206 Singh J. *Medical Profession and Medical Consumer Protection Act*. Available at: www.health library.com/book9_chapter538.htm (accessed 26 August 2011).

207 General Medical Council. *Good Medical Practice*. London: GMC; 2006.

208 Joint Medical Consultative Council/NHS Confederation. *A Clinical Vision of a Reformed NHS*. London: NHS Confederation; July 2007. Available at: www.nhsconfed.org/Publications/Pages/clinicalvision.aspx (accessed 25 September 2011).

209 Picker Institute Europe. *What Patients Need*. Available at: www.pickereurope.org/infoneeds (accessed 20 May 2011).

210 Feest K, Forbes K. *Today's Students, Tomorrow's Doctors: reflections from the wards*. Oxford: Radcliffe Publishing; 2007.

211 The Royal College of General Practitioners and the Health Foundation. *Guiding Patients through Complexity: modern medical generalism*. RCGP, Health Foundation; October 2011. Available at: www.health.org.uk/publications/generalism-report/ (accessed 8 October 2011).

212 Beckford M. Patients need GPs to act like 'local priest'. *Daily Telegraph*. 7 October 2011: 6.

213 Horton R. What's wrong with doctors? *New York Review of Books*. 31 May 2007. Available at: www.nybooks.com/articles/archives/2007/may/31/whats-wrong-with-doctors/?pagination= false (accessed 20 June 2011).

214 Groopman J. *How Doctors Think*. Boston, MA: Houghton Mifflin; 2007.

215 National Association of Primary Care. Sixty step plan to restore faith in NHS. *NAPC News*. 7 December 2011. Available at: www.napc.co.uk/index.php/napc-news-7-december-2011 (accessed 12 January 2012).

Chapter 8: Realising the aims of medicine in the twenty-first century

216 Crisp N. Listen to patients and professionals on the future of the NHS. Letters to the Editor. *The Times*. 26 May 2011; 35.

217 Thursten T. Doctor leading NHS reforms warns of 'tough decisions' over treatment. *Lymington Times*. 17 September 2011: 21.

218 Lewis J. Providers, 'consumers', the state and the delivery of health-care services in twentieth-century Britain. In: Wear A, editor. *Medicine in Society*. 1998. pp. 317–46.

219 Stolberg SG, Pea R. Obama signed health care overhaul bill with a flourish. *New York Times*. 23 March 2010; A19.

220 Duffin J. The impact of single-payer health care on physician income in Canada, 1850–2005. *Am J Public Health*. 2011: **101**(7): 1198–208.

221 Porter R. *The Greatest Benefit to Mankind: a medical history of humanity from antiquity to the present*. 2nd ed. London: Fontana Press; 1997.

222 Collins P. We've named schizophrenia. Now let's treat it. *The Times*. 4 November 2011: 35.

223 Bentall R. *Doctoring the Mind: is our current treatment of mental illness really any good?* New York, NY: New York University Press; 2009.

224 Wipond R. Crisis behind closed doors: antipsychotic drugging of Canada seniors. *Focus Online*. June 2011. Available at: www.mindfreedom.org/kb/psychiatric-drugs/antipsychotics/seniors/canada-seniors-antipsychotic (accessed 20 August 2011).

225 Loveys K. Chemical cosh given to children as young as five. *Daily Mail*. 9 November 2011: 30.

226 Null G, Dean C, Feldman M, *et al*. *Death by Medicine*. Available at: www.webdc.com/pdfs/deathbymedicine.pdf (accessed 20 April 2010).

References

227 Lister S. 'Footprint' that counts cost of NHS care. *The Times*. 12 August 2011: 21.

228 UN Development Reports. *Regional and National Trends in the Human Development Index 1970–2010*. Available at: http://hdr.undp.org/en/data/trends/hybrid/ (accessed 12 June 2011).

229 Cristobal F, Worley P. Transforming health professionals' education. *The Lancet*. 2011; **377**(9773): 1235–6.

230 Keusch GT, Kilama WL, Moon S, *et al*. The global health system: linking knowledge with action; learning from malaria. *PLoS Med*. 2010; **7**(1): e1000193.

231 Porter R. *Blood and Guts: a short history of medicine*. London: Penguin Books; 2002.

232 Tierney WG. Remembrance of things past: trust and the obligations of the intellectual. *Rev High Educ*. 2003; **27**(1): 1–15.

233 Norris TE, Schaad DC, DeWitt D, *et al*. Longitudinal integrated clerkships for medical students: an innovation adopted by medical schools in Australia, Canada, South Africa, and the United States. *Acad Med*. 2009; **84**(7): 902–7.

234 Demarzo MMP, Fontanella BJB, Melo DG, *et al*. Longitudinal medical internship. *Rev Bras Educ Med*. 2010; **34**(3): 430–7.

235 Marchbanks RJ, Good EF. *Complex Neurological and Oto-neurological Remote Care: from space station to clinic*. Paper presented at TeleMed & eHealth 2008, Royal Society of Medicine, London; November 2008.

236 Williams DR, Bashshur RL, Pool SL, *et al*. A strategic vision for telemedicine and medical informatics in space flight. *Telemed J E Health*. 2000; **6**(4): 441–8.

237 Seddon N. The NHS can learn a lot from India … and Scotland. [Opinion] *The Times*. 5 September 2011: 26.

238 Gawande A. *Complications: a surgeon's notes on an imperfect science*. London: Profile Books; 2003.

Chapter 9: 'What's past is prologue': revitalising medical education and training for the twenty-first century

239 Bennet A, Bennet D. Evolution of Organisations: from bureaucracy to intelligent complex adaptive systems. Available at: http://books.google.co.uk/books?hl=en&lr=&id=UDSqNFfzf f0C&oi=fnd&pg=PA5&dq=Evolution+of+Organizations:+from+bureaucracy+to+intelligen t+complex+adaptive+systems.&ots=x_wGvr6JId&sig=5DD83eudr3Eo5u11sSScn7G3AQk #v=onepage&q=Evolution%20of%20Organizations%3A%20from%20bureaucracy%20to%20 intelligent%20complex%20adaptive%20systems.&f=false (accessed 20 January 2007).

240 Collins J, Porras JI. *Built to Last: successful habits of visionary companies*. New York, NY: Harperbusiness; 2004.

241 Welton DN. *Built to Last: successful habits of visionary companies* [summary]. Available at: www.squeezedbooks.com/book/show/20/built-to-last-successful-habits-of-visionary-companies (accessed 20 June 2011).

242 Everley M, Smith J. Making the transition from soft to hard funding: the politics of institutionalizing instructional development programs. *To Improve the Academy*. 1996; **15**: 209–30.

243 Mezirow J. A critical theory of adult learning and education. *Adult Educ*. 1981; **32**(1): 3–24.

244 Bennet A, Bennet D. *The Rise of the Knowledge Organisation: from bureaucracy to intelligent complex adaptive systems*. Available at: http://books.google.co.uk/books?hl=en&lr=&id=UDS qNFfzff0C&oi=fnd&pg=PA5&dq=Evolution+of+Organizations:+from+bureaucracy+to+int elligent+complex+adaptive+systems.&ots=x_wGvr6JId&sig=5DD83eudr3Eo5u11sSScn7G 3AQk#v=onepage&q=Evolution%20of%20Organizations%3A%20from%20bureaucracy%20 to%20intelligent%20complex%20adaptive%20systems.&f=false (accessed 20 January 2007).

245 Wilson V, Pirrie A. *Multidisciplinary Teamworking: beyond the barriers? A review of the Issues*. Scottish Council for Research in Education. Research Report No 96. Edinburgh: SCRE; 2000.

246 Borland S. Doctors ordered to treat old with respect. *Daily Mail*. 1 November 2011: 1.

247 GMC. *What Can You Expect From Your Doctor?* Press Release. 31 October 2011. Available at: www.gmc-uk.org/news/10899.asp (accessed 10 November 2011).

248 Ruiz de Castilla EM. *IAPO: patients' needs must come first*. Press Release. New York, NY: International Alliance of Patients' Organizations: 19 September 2011. Available at: www.epda. eu.com/news/2011-09-19-iapo/ (accessed 28 September 2011).

249 Smith MK. David A. Kolb on experiential learning. *The Encyclopedia of Informal Education*. 2001. Available at: www.ifsociety.org/voxmagister/david_kolb.htm (accessed 24 February 2009).

250 Smith A, Stephens J. *Learning in Clinical Practice: a multidisciplinary approach*. Paper presented at the qualitative Evidence-based Practice Conference, Taking a Critical Stance, Coventry University; 14–16 May 2001.

251 Stigler FL, Duvivier RJ, Weggemans M, *et al.* Health professionals for the 21st century: a students' view. *The Lancet*. 2010; **376**(9756): 1877–8. Available at: www.thelancet.com/journals/lancet/article/PIIS0140-6736%2810%2961968-X/fulltext (accessed 20 May 2011).

252 Cranton P. *Understanding and Promoting Transformative Learning: a guide for educators of adults*. San Francisco, CA: Jossey-Bass; 1994.

253 Hean S, Craddock D, Hammick M. Theoretical insights into interprofessional education: an Association of Medical Educators in Europe guide. *Medical Teacher* (in press).

254 Morrison I. *Flip the Switch*. July 2010. Available at: http://ianmorrison.com/305/ (accessed 20 May 2011).

255 Hood L. A doctor's vision of the future. *Newsweek*. 13 June 2009.

256 www.futuretimeline.net/index.htm

257 Wormald J. *What Will Doctors Be Doing by 2050?* August 2004. Available at: www.gmc-uk. org/Jennifer_Wormald.pdf_25397481.pdf (accessed 7 June 2011).

258 Crisp N. *Turning the World Upside Down: the search for global health in the 21st century*. London: Royal Society of Medicine Press; 2010.

259 Jadad AR, Enkin MW. Computers: transcending our limits? *BMJ*. 2007: **334**(Suppl 1): s8.

260 Fineberg H, Dayrit M, Thibault G, *et al*. Launch panels. Panel 4: strategies for dissemination [Harvard launch of health commission report]. Available at: www.health professionals21.org/index.php/the-report/launch-event (accessed 25 January 2011).

261 Hord S, Rutherford WL, Hulung-Austin L, *et al*. *Taking Charge of Change*. Alexandria, VA: Association for Supervision and Curriculum Development; 1987.

262 Bridges W. *Managing Transitions*. 2nd ed. Philadelphia, PA: Da Capo Press; 2009.

263 Katseva A. *My 'A-ha' Moments at the Business Process Re-engineering Conference: Part 2*. Available at: www.systemscope.com/events/my-%e2%80%9ca-ha%e2%80%9d-moments-at-the-business-process-re-engineering-conference-%e2%80%93-part-2/ (accessed 20 August 2011).

264 Mackinnon LAK. *Book review: Managing Transitions by William Bridges*. Available at: www.think-differently.org/2007/05/book-review-managing-transitions-by/ (accessed 26 March 2008).

265 Rogers EM. *Diffusion of Innovations*. New York, NY: The Free Press; 1995.

266 Evans L, Chauvin S. Faculty developers as change facilitators: the concerns-based model. *To Improve the Academy*. 1993; **12**: 165–78.

267 Loucks-Horsley S. *The Concerns-Based Adoption Model (CBAM): a model for change in individuals*. Dubuque, IA: Kendall/Hunt Publishing; 1996.

268 Isles V, Sutherland K. *Managing Change in the NHS: organisational change; a review for health care managers, professionals and researchers*. London: National Co-ordinating Centre for NHS Service Delivery and Organisation R & D; May 2001. Available at: www.sdo.nihr.ac.uk/files/adhoc/change-management-review.pdf (accessed 20 September 2010).

269 Stockin B. *Initiative and Inertia in the NHS*. London: Nuffield Provincial Hospital Trust; 1995.

270 Slappendel C. Perspectives on innovation in organizations. *Organization Studies*. 1996; **17**(1): 107–29.

271 Katseva A. *My 'A-ha' Moments at the Business Process Re-engineering Conference: Part 1*. Available at: www.systemscope.com/events/my-%E2%80%9Ca-ha%E2%80%9D-moments-at-the-business-process-re-engineering-conference-%E2%80%93-part-1/ (accessed 15 February 2011).

272 Lueddeke GR. Telecommunications in education and training and implications for the communications and information technologies. *Education + Training*. 1997; **39**(6–7): 275–87.

Chapter 10: Facing limitations and challenges: broadening the field of medicine and medical education in the twenty-first century

273 Fisher, S, Crane S, Chaytor, S. *Population Footprints: the UCL–Leverhulme Trust Symposium on Human Population Growth and Global Carrying Capacity.* UCL Policy Briefing, November 2011. Available at: www.ucl.ac.uk/popfootprints/publications/popfoot_policybrief (accessed 15 December 2011).

274 Attenborough D. *Population and Human Development: the key connections.* Available at: www.peopleandplanet.net/?lid=25990&section=33&topic=44 (accessed 15 July 2011).

275 Marian V. FSI and school of medicine expand global health research. *Encina Columns.* 2011: Winter; 1.

276 Collins P. The guardian angels of the NHS are killing it. *The Times* [Opinion]. 10 February 2012: 27.

277 Greenfield S. *You and Me: the neuroscience of identity.* London: Notting Hill Editions; 2011.

278 Kühn S, Romanowski A, Schilling C, *et al.* The neural basis of video gaming. *Translational Psychiatry.* 2011; **1**; e53. Available at: www.nature.com/tp/journal/v1/n11/full/tp201153a.html (accessed 17 November 2011).

279 Green CS, Bavelier D. Action video game modifies visual selective attention. *Nature.* 2003; **423**(6939): 534–7.

280 Rogers RD, Everitt BJ, Baldacchino A, *et al.* Dissociable deficits in the decision-making cognition of chronic amphetamine abusers, opiate abusers, patients with focal damage to prefrontal cortex, and tryptophan-depleted normal volunteers: evidence for monoaminergic mechanisms. *Neuropsychopharmacology.* 1999; **20**(4): 322–39.

281 Celletti F, Reynolds TA, Wright A, *et al.* Educating a new generation of doctors to improve the health of populations in low- and middle-income countries. *PLoS Med.* 2011; **8**(10): e1001108.

282 NHS Confederation. *Feeling Better? Improving patient experience in hospital.* London: NHS Confederation; 2010. Available at: www.nhsconfed.org/Publications/Documents/Feeling_better_Improving_patient_experience_in_hospital_Report.pdf (accessed 27 February 2011).

283 Farmer D. *Strategies for Change: new directions for higher education.* San Francisco, CA: Jossey-Bass; 1990.

284 Dombeck M. *The Medicalization of Mental Illness.* 1 June 2000. Available at: www.mentalhelp.net/poc/view_doc.php?type=doc&id=687 (accessed 15 July 2010).

285 Maben J, Cornwell J, Sweeney K. In praise of compassion. *J Res Nurs.* 2009; **15**(8): 9–13.

286 Hambilton T. *The teachings of Buddha.* Available at: http://home.pacific.net.au/~thambilton/Buddha.html (accessed 17 December 2011).

287 Lyons G. How emerging economies help global growth. *Daily Mail.* 21 November 2011.

288 O'Neill J. *The Growth Map: economic opportunity in the BRICs and beyond.* London: Penguin Books; 2011.

289 Barrows H, Tamblyn, R. *Problem-Based Learning: an approach to medical education.* New York, NY: Springer Publishing; 1980.

290 University of Melbourne Medical School. *Course Attributes.* Available at: www.medicine.unimelb.edu.au/future/md/attributes.html (accessed 10 May 2011).

291 University of Michigan Medical School. *M.D. Program.* Available at: www.med.umich.edu/medschool/edu/md.htm (accessed 18 June 2011).

292 Johns Hopkins Medicine. *Revolution in American Medicine.* Available at: www.hopkinsmedicine.org/about/history/history3.html (accessed 26 September 2011).

293 Stephens C. *Innovations in the University of Southampton's Faculty of Medicine BM Programmes* [email]. 16 February 2012.

294 Playdon Z-J, Josephy A, editors. *Journeys in Postgraduate Medical Education.* London: Third Space Press; 2011.

295 Kent, Surrey & Sussex Postgraduate Deanery. *GEAR: graduate education and assessment regulations.* London: KSS; 2011.

296 Chen YF, Chen L. Views from Asia – retaining Flexner's essence while transforming education. Available at: http://healthprofessionals21.org/index.php/news-a-events/100-viewpoint-y-f-chen (accessed 12 January 2012).

297 The George Washington University Medical Centre, University of Pretoria and the Bill & Melinda Gates Foundation. *The Sub-Saharan African Medical School Study: data, observation and opportunity.* Available at: http://samss.org/samss.upload/documents/126.pdf (accessed 4 March 2012).

298 Social Care Institute for Excellence. *Dignity in Care: the dignity factors.* Available at: www.scie.org.uk/publications/guides/guide15/index.asp# (accessed 17 September 2011).

299 Department of Health. Government accepts new recommendations from NHS. Available at: www.dh.gov.uk/health/2012/01/forum-response/ (accessed 14 January 2012).

300 Fineberg HV. Health reform beyond health insurance. Available at: http://iom.edu/Global/News%20Announcements/Health-Reform-Beyond-Health-Insurance.aspx (accessed 20 October 2011).

301 World Overpopulation: awareness, sustainability, carrying capacity, and overconsumption. Available at: www.overpopulation.org/solutions.html (accessed 8 December 2011).

302 Le Fanu J. *The Rise and Fall of Modern Medicine.* London: Hachette Digital, Little, Brown Book Group; 2011.

303 Sharp P. *The NHS in the next decade.* London: Centre for Workforce Intelligence (CfWI); 2011.

304 Stanford University, Centre for compassion and altruism research and education. *Research Projects.* Available at: http://ccare.stanford.edu/programs/research-projects (accessed 15 October 2011).

305 The College of Medicine. *The Crisis in Caring.* Available at: www.collegeofmedicine.org.uk/crisis-caring (accessed 9 January 2012).

306 Kendall P. How to help the aged. *Seven magazine. The Sunday Telegraph.* 29 January 2012: 15.

307 Sharp P. *Reviewing and Comparing Recent Developments in National Health Workforce Planning: patient pathways models (UK).* London: Centre for Workforce Intelligence (CfWI); 8 September 2011.

308 Centre for Workforce Intelligence (CfWI). *Horizontal Scanning at CfWI.* London: CfWI: 2011.

309 Torjeson I. NHS is set to train 60% more consultants than needed by 2020. Available at: http://careers.bmj.com/careers/advice/view-article.html?id=20006582 (accessed 11 February 2012).

310 Medical Education England (MEE). *Better Training Better Care.* Available at: www.mee.nhs.uk/our_work/work_priorities/better_training_better_care.aspx (accessed 25 October 2011).

311 Horton R. *A New Epoch for Health Professionals' Education.* Available at: http://healthprofessionals21.org/index.php/the-report/comments/26-a-new-epoch-for-health-professionals-education-richard-horton (accessed 20 February 2012).

312 Snyder J, Dharamsi S, Crooks VA. Fly-By medical care: conceptualising the global and local social responsibilities of medical tourists and physician voluntourists. Available at: www.globalizationandhealth.com/content/7/1/6 (accessed 20 October 2011).

313 British Medical Association. Core professional values. Available at: www.bma.org.uk/health care_policy/professional_values/profval.jsp?page=3 (accessed 20 July 2008).

314 Sagan C. Pale blue dot: a vision of the human future in space. 1st ed. New York: Ballantine Books; 1997 (brief video: www.youtube.com/watch?v=p86BPM1GV8M).

References

Epilogue

315 Dickson G. Transformations in Canadian health systems leadership: an analytical perspective. *Leadership in Health Services*. 2009; **22**(4): 292–305.

316 Oandasan I, Baker GR, Barker K, *et al. Teamwork in Healthcare: promoting effective teamwork in healthcare in Canada*. Ottawa, ON: Canadian Health Services Research Foundation; 2006.

317 The Canadian Health Leadership Network (CHLNet): CHLNet's Value proposition. Available at: www.chlnet.ca/ (accessed 28 February 2012).

318 McLean K, *et al*. Clinical Advice & Leadership: a report from the NHS Future Forum (13 June 2011). Available at: www.gponline.com/News/article/1074776/download-nhs-future-forum-clinical-advice-leadership-report/ (accessed 28 February 2012).

319 Collins J. *Good to Great and the Social Sectors: why business thinking is not the answer*. Boulder, CO: J Collins; 2005.

Index

Note: references to figures and tables are in **bold**.

Index